AF710386

Neuroregulatory Mechanisms in Aging

Pergamon studies in neuroscience No 8

Series editor Dr William Winlow, *Dept. of Physiology, University of Leeds, LS2 9NQ, UK*

Neuroscience is one of the major growth areas in the biological sciences and draws both techniques and ideas from many other scientific disciplines. *Pergamon studies in neuroscience* presents both monographs and multi-author volumes drawn from the whole range of the subject and brings together the subdisciplines that have arisen from the recent explosive development of the neurosciences.

Pergamon studies in neuroscience includes contributions from molecular and cellular neurobiology, developmental neuroscience (including tissue culture), neural networks and systems research (both clinical and basic) and behavioural neuroscience (including ethology). The series is designed to appeal to research workers in clinical and basic neuroscience, their graduate students and advanced undergraduates with an interest in the subject.

1. **Function and dysfunction in the basal ganglia** *ed.* A. J. Franks, J. W. Ironside, R. H. S. Mindham, R. J. Smith, E. G. S. Spokes *and* W. Winlow

2. **Comparative aspects of neuropeptide function** *ed.* Ernst Florey *and* George B. Stefano

3. **Neuromuscular transmission: basic and applied aspects** *ed.* Angela Vincent *and* Dennis Wray

4. **Neurobiology of motor programme selection: new approaches to the study of behavioural choose** *ed.* Jenny Kien, Catherine R. McCrohan *and* William Winlow

5. **Interleukin-1 in the brain** *ed.* Nancy J. Rothwell *and* Robert D. Dantzer

New in 1993

A theory of the striatum J. Wickens
Glycobiology and the brain *ed.* M. Nicolini and P. F. Zatta
Neural modeling and neural networks *ed.* F. Ventriglia
Neurophysiology of ingestion *ed.* D. A. Booth
Neuroregulatory mechanisms in aging *ed.* Maynard H. Makman and George B. Stefano
Thalamic networks for relay and modulation *ed.* Diego Minciacchi, Marco Molinari, Giorgio Macchi and Edward G. Jones

Neuroregulatory Mechanisms in Aging

edited by

Maynard H. Makman and George B. Stefano

PERGAMON PRESS

OXFORD · NEW YORK · SEOUL · TOKYO

U.K.	Pergamon Press Ltd, Headington Hill Hall, Oxford OX3 0BW, England
U.S.A.	Pergamon Press, Inc., 660 White Plains Road, Tarrytown, New York 10591-5153, U.S.A.
KOREA	Pergamon Press Korea, KPO Box 315, Seoul 110-603, Korea
JAPAN	Pergamon Press Japan, Tsunashima Building Annex, 3-20-12 Yushima, Bunkyoku, Tokyo 113, Japan

Copyright © 1993 Pergamon Press Ltd

All Rights Reserved. No part of this publication may be reproduced, stored in a retrieval system or transmitted in any form or by any means: electronic, electrostatic, magnetic tape, mechanical, photocopying, recording or otherwise, without permission in writing from the publishers.

QP 356.25 .N48 1993

First edition 1993

Library of Congress Cataloging in Publication Data

A catalogue record for this book is available from the Library of Congress

British Library Cataloguing in Publication Data

A catalogue record for this book is available from the British Library

ISBN 0 08 041989 5

In order to make this volume available as economically and as rapidly as possible it has been produced by translation from the authors' word processor disks. Every effort has been made to ensure an exact reproduction within the time available.

Printed in Great Britain by BPCC Wheatons Ltd, Exeter

Contents

List of Contributors

S. BHATNAGAR
Aging Research Program, McGill University-Douglas Hospital Research Center, Departments of Psychiatry, Neurology and Neurosurgery and Experimental Medicine, McGill University, Montreal, Canada

T. V. BILFINGER
Department of Surgery, Health Science Center, University Hospital, SUNY at Stony Brook, Stony Brook, NY 11794, USA

P. BLANCO
Departamento de Biología Molecular (CSIC-UAM), Universidad Autónoma, Canto Blanco, 28049 Madrid, Spain

R. J. BODNAR
Department of Psychology, Queens College, Flushing, New York, USA

S. R. BODNOFF
Aging Research Program, McGill University-Douglas Hospital Research Center, Departments of Psychiatry, Neurology and Neurosurgery and Experimental Medicine, McGill University, Montreal, Canada

E. BOGONEZ
Departamento de Biología Molecular (CSIC-UAM), Universidad Autónoma, Canto Blanco, 28049 Madrid, Spain

D. O. CARPENTER
Wadsworth Center for Laboratories and Research, New York State Department of Health and School of Public Health, Albany, New York 12201-0509, USA

E. E. EL-FAKAHANY
Department of Pharmacology and Toxicology, University of Maryland, School of Pharmacy, Baltimore, MD 21201, USA

G. L. FRICCHIONE
Brigham's Womens Hospital, Division of Psychiatry, Harvard Medical School, Boston, Mass., USA

I. HIROTSU
Laboratory of Experimental Pharmacology, Suntory Institute for Biomedical Research, 1-1-1, Wakayamadai, Shimamoto-Cho, Mishima-Gun, Osaka 618, Japan

N. HORI
Wadsworth Center for Laboratories and Research, New York State Department of Health and School of Public Health, Albany, New York 12201-0509, USA and Department of Pharmacology, Faculty of Dentistry, Kyushu University, 1-1-3, Maidashi, Higashi-Ku, Fukuoka 812, Japan

C. JANSE
Department of Biology, Vrije Universiteit, 1007 MC, Amsterdam, The Netherlands

J. A. JOSEPH
Molecular Physiology and Genetics Section, Gerontology Research Center/NIA, Baltimore, MD 21224, USA

N. KATSUDA
Department of Pharmacology, Faculty of Dentistry, Kyushu University, 1-1-3, Maidashi, Higashi-Ku, Fukuoka 812, Japan

M. H. MAKMAN
Departments of Biochemistry and Molecular Pharmacology, Albert Einstein College of Medicine, Bronx, New York 10461, USA

L. MALLOZZI
Multidisciplinary Center for the Study of Aging, State University of New York/College at Old Westbury, Old Westbury, New York 11568, USA

A. MARTÍNEZ-SERRANO
Departamento de Biología Molecular (CSIC-UAM), Universidad Autónoma, Canto Blanco, 28049 Madrid, Spain

M. J. MEANEY
Aging Research Program, McGill University-Douglas Hospital Research Center, Departments of Psychiatry, Neurology and Neurosurgery and Experimental Medicine, McGill University, Montreal, Canada

D. O'DONNELL
Aging Research Program, McGill University-Douglas Hospital Research Center, Departments of Psychiatry, Neurology and Neurosurgery and Experimental Medicine, McGill University, Montreal, Canada

G. W. PASTERNAK
The George C. Cotias Laboratory of Neuro-Oncology, Memorial Sloan-Kettering Cancer Center and Department of Neurology and Neuroscience, Department of Pharmacology, Cornell University Medical College, New York 10021, USA

J. POIRIER
Aging Research Program, McGill University-Douglas Hospital Research Center, Departments of Psychiatry, Neurology and Neurosurgery and Experimental Medicine, McGill University, Montreal, Canada

S. PRYOR
Multidisciplinary Center for the Study of Aging, State University of New York/College at Old Westbury, Old Westbury, New York 11568, USA

P. G. PUERTAS
Departamento de Biología Molecular (CSIC-UAM), Universidad Autónoma, Canto Blanco, 28049 Madrid, Spain

J. SATRÚSTEGUI
Departamento de Biología Molecular (CSIC-UAM), Universidad Autónoma, Canto Blanco, 28049 Madrid, Spain

G. B. STEFANO
Old Westbury Neuroscience Institute and Multidisciplinary Center for the Study of Aging, State University of New York/College at Old Westbury, New York 11568-0210, USA

M. VILLALBA
Departamento de Biología Molecular (CSIC-UAM), Universidad Autónoma, Canto Blanco, 28049 Madrid, Spain

S. A. WELNER
Aging Research Program, McGill University-Douglas Hospital Research Center, Departments of Psychiatry, Neurology and Neurosurgery and Experimental Medicine, McGill University, Montreal, Canada

Introduction and Perspectives on the Neurobiology of Aging

MAYNARD H. MAKMAN[1] and GEORGE B. STEFANO[2]

[1] *Departments of Biochemistry and Molecular Pharmacology, Albert Einstein College of Medicine, Bronx, New York 10461, USA*
[2] *Old Westbury Neuroscience Institute and Multidisciplinary Center for the Study of Aging, State University of New York/ College at Old Westbury, New York 11568-0210, USA*

Studies of aging have generally been concerned with determinants of life span and cause of death, decreases in proliferative capacity of different cell types, and functional impairments associated with old age. An additional major consideration, of particular relevance to aging of the nervous system, is the existence of and interaction between "normal" aging and specific disease states that are more likely to occur with increased age. The nature and extent of changes that occur with increasing age may differ considerably in different species and also in the various organs or tissues of a given species. Functionally important age-related changes may or may not also be important causes of death of the animal. In addition, a particular age-related pathological process may be unique to one species or to a group of animal species. On the other hand, important features of senescence may be shared by different animals, and indeed there may be aspects of aging that are shared by both vertebrate and invertebrate species.

There may be certain animals that do not appear to age, e.g., certain paramecia and bivalve molluscs. However, it is possible that even those animals age, but they also have an extremely long natural life span. We may not see each individual organism age simply because of the occurrence of accidental death. The concept of negative pleiotropy has been employed to account for biological senescence. Indeed, cumulative and unavoidable events or reactions may eventually lead to decrements in function and/or death of an organism. Hence, oxygen-free radicals, advanced glycosylation endproducts, protein adducts, damage occurring with genetic repair, etc., may accumulate to critical levels at which normal functions are compromised.

Furthermore, the causative factor may even be a once useful process now occurring in excess. Over time molecular alterations may pyramid into cellular, tissue, organ and organismal modifications /compensations whereby an individual will exhibit a general decline in function and reactive capacity. Such age-associated modifications, at least certain of them, are essentially inevitable. Also, by such processes alterations that continue to occur may eventually allow the organism to succumb to an environmental assault which at an earlier time posed no threat. Thus, the aging process may insure for enhanced vulnerability and death of a particular organism, thereby allowing for turnover of the population and the possibility for incorporation of useful mutations into the population.

In the human population there is evidence of age-related decrements in central nervous system (CNS) function, including behavioral impairment and altered response to CNS drugs. Certain of these decrements may apply to the general human population and be due to selective age-related alterations in neurotransmitter systems that also occur with aging in other mammalian species. However, there may be no close counterpart in other species to senile dementia of the Alzheimer's type, a human disease associated with, and possibly caused by, loss of certain central cholinergic neurons. It is often difficult to be certain in studies of human aging whether or not particular age-related changes represent "normal" aging due to factors intrinsic to the organism or unavoidable interactions with the environment, or to specific disease processes that may be as yet undefined. However, it appears likely, based on animal studies, that age-associated changes in CNS neurotransmitter systems indeed occur independent of any specific disease process. These changes may be manifest in altered function *per se*, altered functional "reserves" and/or altered predisposition to or severity of pathological processes.

Not all functional components or neuronal cell types are affected similarly by the aging process. Probably in most instances the underlying cause(s) for a particular change is (are) not known. The degree of plasticity of the adult nervous system is only now beginning to be appreciated. Also, the possible regenerative capacity in some situations remains to be evaluated. Additionally, changes in these parameters with aging remain to be investigated.

The chapters in this book present studies of neuronal aging in a variety of species. Also, a variety of approaches are utilized in order to gain insight into the nature and significance of age-related changes. The overall intent is to present some indication of the wide scope of these studies, to give some idea of the present state of knowledge of the neurobiology of aging in selected areas, and to include representative examples of approaches and "model systems" for such studies. We believe the comparative biological aspect to be of particular importance. The comparative study of neuronal aging greatly enhances our knowledge of the functioning of animal species that may be quite different from one another, yet contain nervous systems with many similarities with respect to their transmitter systems as well as the basic sensory, motor and integrative functions. These studies reveal surprising similarities in the integrative processes regulating function and the life cycle in mammals and invertebrates. Comparative studies of neuronal aging may also serve to focus attention on those aspects of neuronal processes and adaptive mechanisms that are necessary for survival and propagation of the organism. For these reasons, such studies have a general relevance to our understanding of life cycle events and the aging process in all living organisms.

Since molecular biology has not yet provided the means for intervention in the aging process, at present we are left with the pharmacological approach to alleviate some of the effects of aging and to restore age-associated alterations of normal function. Given the vast amount of information that has been accumulated concerning the pharmacology of the nervous system, it becomes important to attempt to use this information to intervene appropriately in the aging process. Also, age-related changes in the responses of humans to CNS-active drugs have provided significant clues to the possible underlying changes in the nervous system that occur with age. For these reasons, neuropharmacological studies have provided a major focus for this book.

Clearly, the nervous system plays a central role in the integrative dynamic responsiveness of the organism. At the cellular and molecular levels, modifications associated with damage or aging can be masked by a host of compensatory mechanisms. However, once the utilization of a particular compensatory mechanism reaches a point at which no further change in the mechanism is possible or at which no further response of the organism to that mechanism is possible, then the functioning of the organism is compromised. A characteristic feature of aging appears to be an altered, generally decreased, intrinsic or adaptive response, including decreased reliability of homeostatic regulation. In this regard, the role of the nervous system is particularly important since it may be the first system to "signal" a decrease in the dynamic capacity to respond.

The integrative functions of the nervous system include not only the obvious hard wiring, including direct innervation of peripheral tissues, but also a sort of soft wiring that allows for bidirectional communication between systems. Examples of the latter include not only the neuroendocrine system but, as has become increasingly evident in recent years, the immune system. These interactions are considered in the present volume in relation to the neurobiology of aging.

What concerns us as cognitive beings is that the quality of our life, as we age, should be such that we can continue to function with dignity. With that in mind, the importance of the continued function of our integrative mechanisms is self evident. Of these mechanisms, none is more important than the nervous system, that which brings together intellectual and spiritual as well as bodily functions.

The Effects of Acetylcholine and Aging on Electrical Excitability of the Central Nervous System

D. O. CARPENTER[1,4], I. HIROTSU[2], N. KATSUDA[3] and N. HORI[1,3]

[1] *Wadsworth Center for Laboratories and Research, New York State Department of Health and School of Public Health, Albany, NY 12201-0509, USA*
[2] *Laboratory of Experimental Pharmacology, Suntory Institute for Biomedical Research, 1-1-1, Wakayamadai, Shimamoto-Cho, Mishima-Gun, Osaka 618, Japan*
[3] *Department of Pharmacology, Faculty of Dentistry, Kyushu University, 1-1-3, Maidashi, Higashi-Ku, Fukuoka 812, Japan*
[4] *To whom correspondence should be addressed*

Introduction

Acetylcholine may be only one of a large number of neurotransmitter substances within the mammalian central nervous system, but increasingly it is understood to play a particularly important role in normal neuronal functioning and particularly in such complex functions as learning and memory (Kopelman, 1986; Deutsch, 1971). Furthermore, disruptions of this normal functioning appear to be very important, and may be the etiologic factor of prime significance, in abnormal aging of the nervous system, as in Alzheimer's disease.

As in the peripheral nervous systems there are both nicotinic and muscarinic acetylcholine receptors in mammalian brain, and activation of these receptors leads to both excitatory and inhibitory responses (Kelly *et al.*, 1979). Muscarinic receptors predominate, and the most common response to acetylcholine application is a depolarization resulting from a decrease in K^+ conductance, which gives rise to a prolonged excitation (Krnjevic and Phillis, 1963; Spehlmann, 1963).

The functional significance of muscarinic acetylcholine receptors in mammalian central nervous system is indicated both by demonstration of memory facilitation when animals are treated with anticholinesterases (Deutsch, 1971) and of deficits in short-term memory when humans or animals are given receptor antagonists that resemble those seen in normal human aging (Glick *et al.*, 1973; Drachman and Leavitt, 1974; Peterson, 1977; Elrod and Buccafusco, 1988). Deficits of short-term memory are characteristic of normal aging to a degree, and are a major indicator of the onset of Alzheimer's disease even before there is a general loss of cognitive function (Crystal *et al.*, 1988). In both animals (Smith, 1988) and man (Bartus *et al.*, 1982) dysfunction of cholinergic systems has been correlated with deficits of short-term memory. There is a particular loss of cholinergic innervation of the cortex in Alzheimer's disease (Davis and Mahoney, 1976; Whitehouse *et al.*, 1981). While the etiology of Alzheimer's disease remains a subject of some dispute (Palmer and Gershon, 1990), one of the major hypotheses is that the disease may actually be a result of the loss of cholinergic neurons (Coyle *et al.*, 1983). Whether or not the loss of cholinergic neurons is the cause or only one symptom of a more general loss of neurons (cf. Maragos *et al.*, 1987), it is clear that loss of cholinergic innervation contributes to the symptomology of the disease. Although there is no satisfactory treatment for the disease, the only drug therapies which have been shown to provide at least symptomatic improvement is use of cholinesterase inhibitors (Summers *et al.*, 1986; Harbaugh *et al.*, 1984; Brinkman and Gershon, 1983; Christie *et al.*, 1981; Becker and Giacobini, 1988).

In this chapter we will review a variety of results obtained in our laboratories by use of brain slices from rats of different ages. We have performed a series of studies investigating the effects of aging on electrophysiologic indicators of learning and memory, and other studies on the responses to acetylcholine application and the effects of activation of these muscarinic receptors on general neuronal excitability as well as on indicators of learning and memory. The goal of these studies is to understand the neurophysiologic and neurochemical basis of the decremental changes in the central nervous system in both normal aging and in diseases such as Alzheimer's where there is a selective neuronal loss.

Methods

Experiments were performed on slices of rat brain obtained from either hippocampus or piriform cortex using methods previously described (ffrench-Mullen *et al.*, 1983; Hori *et al.*, 1988; Hirotsu *et al.*, 1989). Most experiments were performed on young male Wistar rats (approximately 2 months of age and 250-300 gm), but some studies used young (2 months), middle-aged (12 months) or old (24 months) Fisher rats (about 300 gm). General techniques involved quick removal of the brain after cervical dislocation of the animal, blocking of the brain so as to allow sectioning by slices (400-450 μm diameter) using a vibrotome and incubation of the slices for a period of at least 1 hr at 35°C. The slices were then removed to the recording chamber, mounted under a nylon net and submerged and perfused (2-3 ml/min) with an artificial Krebs-Ringer solution with the composition (in mM) NaCl, 124; KCl, 5; $KHPO_4$, 1.24; $CaCl_2$-$2H_2O$, 2.4; $MgSO_4$-$7H_2O$, 1.3; $NaHCO_3$, 26 and D-glucose, 10, pH 7.4.

Three types of recordings were made: population recordings of field potentials evoked upon stimulation of synaptic pathways, extracellular recordings of single neuronal activity and intracellular recordings from pyramidal neurons of either hippocampus (CA1) or piriform cortex. Population recordings were made using glass microelectrodes (tip resistance 1-6 MΩ) filled with 2 M sodium chloride or normal Krebs-Ringer, while for intracellular recordings electrodes had resistances of 80-100 MΩ and were filled with potassium acetate.

Electrical stimulation was delivered through a monopolar stainless-steel electrode (250 μm tip diameter) positioned either on the Schaffer-commissural fiber system in CA3 in hippocampus or on the lateral olfactory tract (LOT) in piriform cortex. The routine frequency of activation of the synaptic pathways was 0.2 Hz, using a 50-μs duration pulse at a current intensity capable of evoking a population spike of approximately 40% maximal response. When it was desired to elicit long-term potentiation, a tetanus of 200 Hz was applied for 1 sec. After tetanic stimulation, ten consecutive responses were averaged at each time point. Membrane resistance was measured by passing current through the recording electrode via a bridge circuit.

Procedures of ionophoretic application of acetylcholine and other transmitters have been previously described (ffrench-Mullen *et al.*, 1983; Hori *et al.*, 1988). Ionophoretic electrodes (3-7 barrels) were filled with various combinations of 1 M acetylcholine chloride, pH 3-4 (Sigma), 1 M sodium glutamate (Aldrich or Katayama); 1 M L-aspartate (K&K or Wako), 1 M homocysteate acid (Sigma) 0.1 M N-methyl-D-aspartate (Sigma) or 10 mM quisqualic acid (Sigma) in 150 mM NaCl. Antagonists of transmitter actions and acetylcholinesterase inhibitors were added to the perfusion and applied to the bath. These substances included scopolamine (Nakarai Chemicals, Kyota), atropine (Sigma), bicuculline chloride (Torris), tetrahydroaminoacridine (THA) (Yoshitomi) and strychnine (Sigma).

Results: changes in neuronal responsiveness and in long-term potentiation with aging

Figure 1 illustrates changes in the amplitudes of electrical responses elicited by activation of normal synaptic pathways in rat hippocampal slices as a function of age. These recordings were made in hippocampal area CA1, a region known to be associated with learning and memory. The traces show representative responses from a young (2 months) and old (24 months) animal at fast (upper) and slow (lower) sweep speed. There are at least three major waves. The initial brief negative-going (downward) deflection is an artifact resulting from the electrical stimulation of the synaptic input via the Schaffer collateral pathway, coming from area CA3 of the hippocampus, and has no physiological significance. The second negative-going peak, most apparent in the fast sweeps and occurring at a latency of about 2 msec after the stimulus, reflects the population recording of the excitatory post-synaptic potentials (EPSPs) in the CA1 pyramidal neurons. The irregularities on the falling phase of the response result from the discharge of the post-synaptic neurons. Sometimes this discharge is relatively synchronous, in which case there is a distinct notch on the falling phase of the potential. In other cases, the discharge is more synchronous and appears only as irregularities on the falling phase. Following this peak there is a slow, positive-going peak, seen more clearly in the slower sweep recordings at the bottom of the EPSPs.

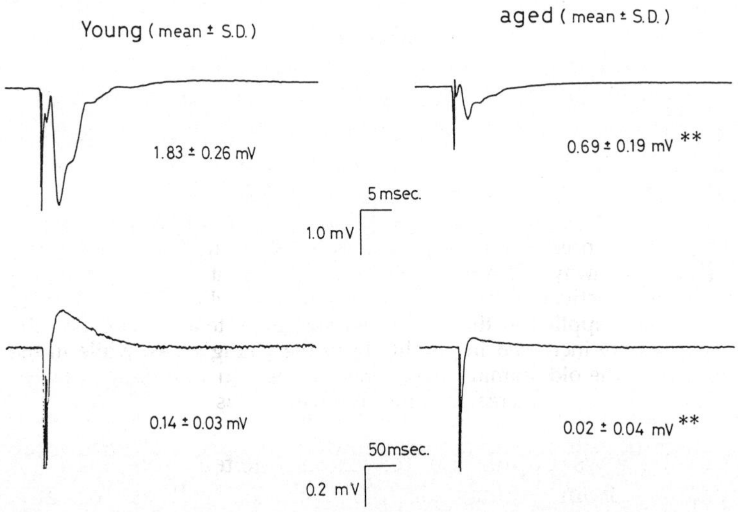

FIG. 1. Electrical recordings of population EPSPs recorded in rat hippocampus CA1 upon stimulation of the Schaffer collateral pathway recorded in young (about 2 months) and old (about 24 months) animals. The means and standard deviations represent data from 29 and 6 animals, respectively. The upper traces are at faster sweep to show the initial monosynaptic excitatory component (the second negative wave), while the lower traces are at slower speed to show the later positive component.

The major difference in responses from young and old animals is that the amplitude is much less in old animals. When such recordings were made from many slices, the mean peak amplitude in slices from young animals was 1.83 ± 0.25 mV, while a similar sample from a 24-month animal (which is very old for a rat) was 0.69 ± 0.19 mV. The lower traces at slower sweep show that the late, slow after hyperpolarization (the positive-going component), is equally larger in young animals. Although there may be some other factors which contribute to these differences (such as the nature of the connective tissue around the neurons), these observations suggest that neurons from young animals are much more responsive than those from old animals.

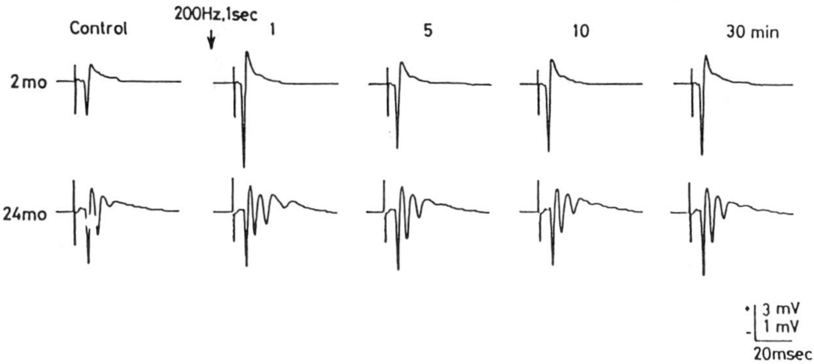

FIG. 2. Responses recorded in CA1 upon stimulation of the Schaffer collateral pathway in 2-month and 24-month-old rats. The response to a single pulse activation is shown at the left, after which a 1 sec, 200 Hz tetanus was applied at the arrow. Following the tetanic activation the responses are increased in amplitude in the young slices, while in the slices from the old animals there is less increase in amplitude but clear increases in the later waveforms.

Figure 2 shows population responses elicited from area CA1 of hippocampus from young and old rats, as well as the effect of application of a 200-Hz tetanic stimulation of the Schaffer collateral pathway. In young animals, the synaptic response shows a single peak and is large relative to that in the old animals, as already shown in Figure 1. In addition to being smaller in amplitude, the response to a similar stimulation of old animals shows one or more additional peaks of response, reflecting a more prolonged excitation.

When a tetanic stimulation is applied to this pathway both a transient and prolonged change in excitability is induced. Immediately after stimulation, there is a post-tetanic potentiation (PTP), which results from an increase in transmitter release from presynaptic terminals, probably as a result of an increase in terminal entry or mobilization of calcium (Nussinovitch and Rahamimoff, 1988). PTP is characteristic of almost all synapses. At some synapses, including this, there is a more long-lasting potentiation called long-term potentiation (LTP). This is apparent as a prolonged and perhaps permanent increase in the excitability of the synapse. While the PTP is maximal within seconds at the end of the tetanic stimulation, LTP is maintained for the duration of a brain slice experiment and may, in fact, be a permanent change in synaptic excitability (Kuba and Kumamoto, 1990). For this reason, LTP is widely considered to be an electrophysiological indicator of prolonged or indefinite synaptic plasticity, and the best available model of learning and memory studied with electrophysiological methods.

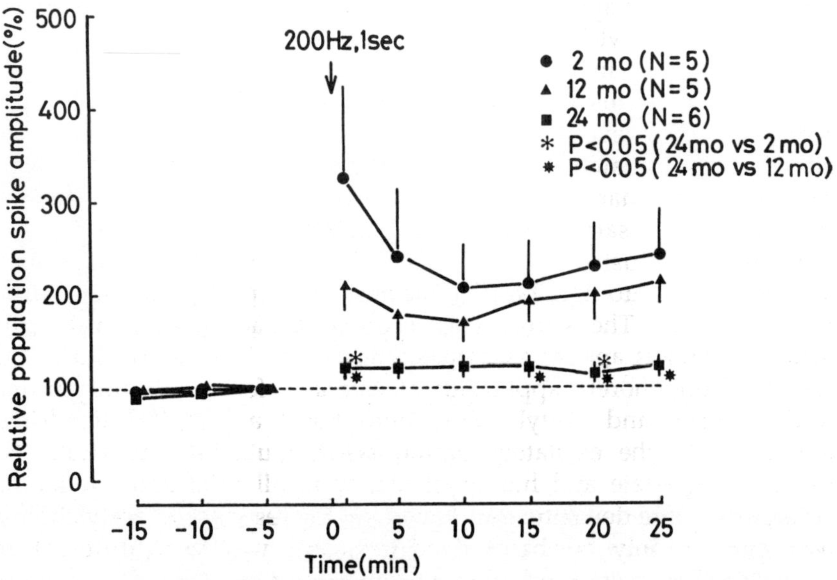

FIG 3. Plot of peak amplitude of population EPSPs with time recorded following tetanic stimulation (200 Hz, 1 sec) of the Schaffer collateral pathway in young (2 months), middle-aged (12 months) and old (24 months) rats. The early PTP decays show the underlying LTP in all but the old animals. Each point represents the means ± S.E.M.

Figure 3 is a plot of the mean amplitudes of PTP and LTP as a function of control values prior to tetanic stimulation in 2-month, 12-month and 24-month Fisher rats. The results of Figure 3 indicate that both PTP and LTP are much more pronounced in slices from the young animals. At 12 months the LTP is still prominent, but at 24 months there is essentially no PTP and only a small LTP. In the old animals, the degree of potentiation is much less at all time points, although the same processes appear to be present, as indicated by smaller increases in the amplitude of the first peak as well as an increase in the number and sizes of the latter peaks. These results are consistent with the view that LTP is a reflection of the ability of plasticity of the nervous system, and that such plasticity is reduced as a part of the normal aging process.

There is a considerable body of evidence indicating that the transmitter at this synapse is an excitatory amino acid (Collingridge *et al.*, 1983). At several, but not all, sites in mammalian brain, LTP is prevented by treatment with antagonists of NMDA receptors, one of the several types of excitatory amino acid receptors. This is the case at this particular synapse (Wigström *et al.*, 1986). However, antagonists of muscarinic acetylcholine receptors also influence the development of LTP, as is shown in Figure 4. When scopolamine was applied before the tetanic stimulus at 10^{-5}M, both PTP and LTP were significantly reduced. If, however, the scopolamine was applied after LTP had already been initiated (lower plot) there was no obvious effect. These results suggest that a normal functioning of muscarinic acetylcholine receptors is necessary for LTP generation but not for maintenance.

Figure 5 illustrates the effects of ionophoretically applied acetylcholine onto the basal dendrites of a pyramidal neuron in piriform cortex. The neuron was recorded extracellularly, so that the action potentials appear as biphasic responses. The figure shows the results of ionophoretic application of several different excitatory amino acid agonists and acetylcholine onto basal and apical dendrites. Responses to the excitatory amino acids, glutamate, aspartate, N-methyl-D-aspartate and homocysteate, were all brief and similar on both parts of the dendritic tree. However, the response to acetylcholine was present only on basal dendrites, and was very different in character. This response had a relatively long latency, and was very prolonged, lasting for about 6 sec.

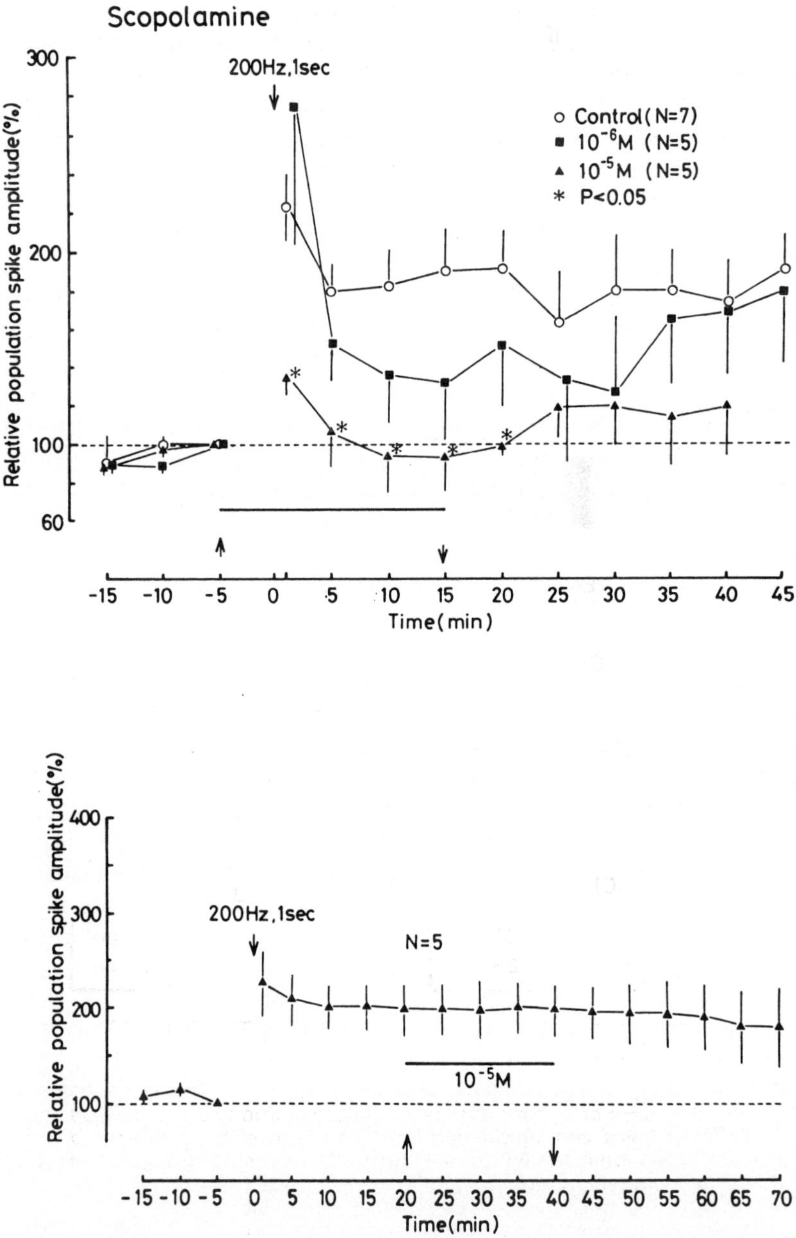

FIG. 4. Effects of scopolamine on LTP in CA1. Scopolamine was applied from 5 min before to 15 min after the tetanus (A) or 20-40 min after the tetanus (B). Each point represents the mean ± S.E.M. (From Hirotsu *et al.*, 1989; used with permission).

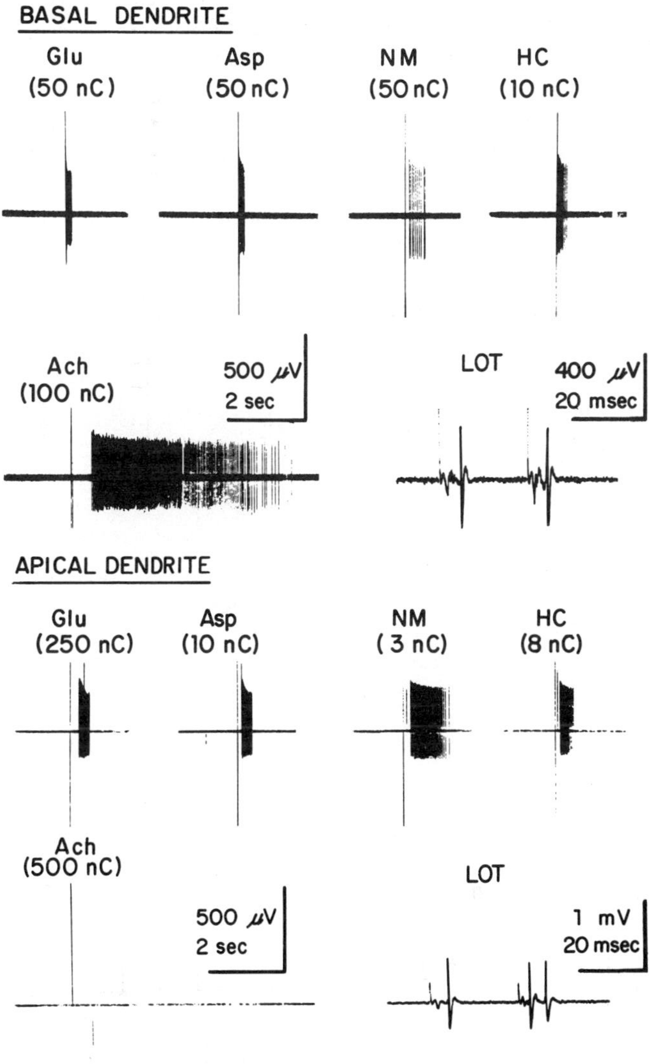

FIG. 5. Pattern of responses to the excitatory amino acid transmitters and ACh on basal and apical dendrites of a neuron of piriform cortex. Recordings are made with extracellular electrodes. From the cut surface the ionophoretic electrode was 50 µm deep for the basal and 300 µm deep for the apical recordings. Although the relative sensitivities of the amino acid responses are not the same at the two sites, there are brisk responses at both places. ACh produces a delayed but prolonged excitation of the basal dendrites, but is without effect on apical dendrites. Glu, glutamate; Asp, aspartate; NM, NMDA; and HC, homocysteic acid. (From ffrench-Mullen *et al.*, 1983; used with permission.)

The muscarinic acetylcholine response on mammalian central neurons has been described in elegant detail by Brown and Adams (1980) and their colleagues (Adams *et al.*, 1982), and that in both hippocampus and piriform cortex is similar to what they describe. They called the ion channel on which acetylcholine acts the "M" channel (for muscarine). It is a voltage-dependent K^+ channel that is *closed* by acetylcholine. This K^+ channel is normally closed at potentials more negative than about –60 mV, but opens at more depolarized potentials. Since the resting membrane potential of many central neurons is close to this value, the M channel is normally opened when the neuron is depolarized by excitatory synaptic events, and this has the result of counteracting the depolarizing stimulus. Consequently, the opening of M channels tends to reduce repetitive discharge.

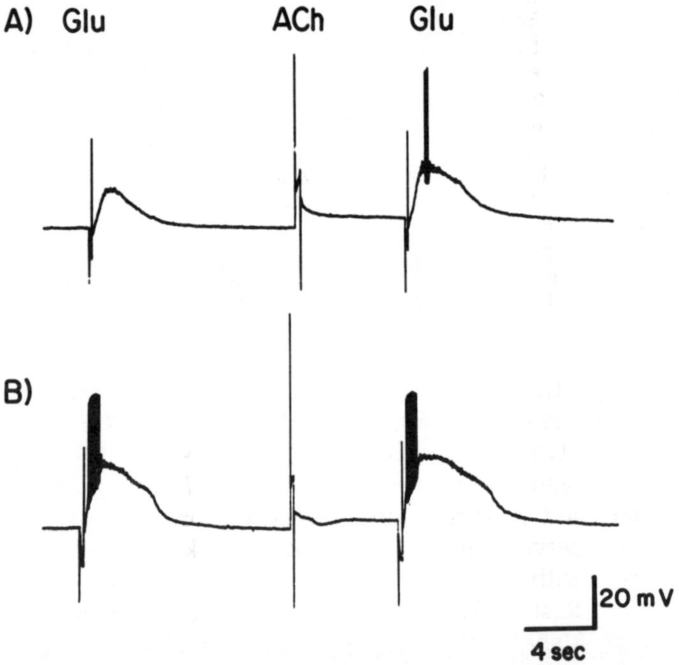

FIG. 6. Potentiation by Ach of a response to glutamate (Glu), from an intracellular recording of a pyramidal neuron in piriform cortex. (A) Glutamate was applied at 100 nC and ACh at 400 nC. (B) Glutamate was applied at 200 nC. Ionophoresis was at the cut surface on the basal dendrites. Membrane potential was –65 mV. The ACh application did not by itself induce discharge of the neuron. There is some distortion of the spike amplitudes due to the time constant of the recording system. (From ffrench-Mullen *et al.*, 1983; used with permission.)

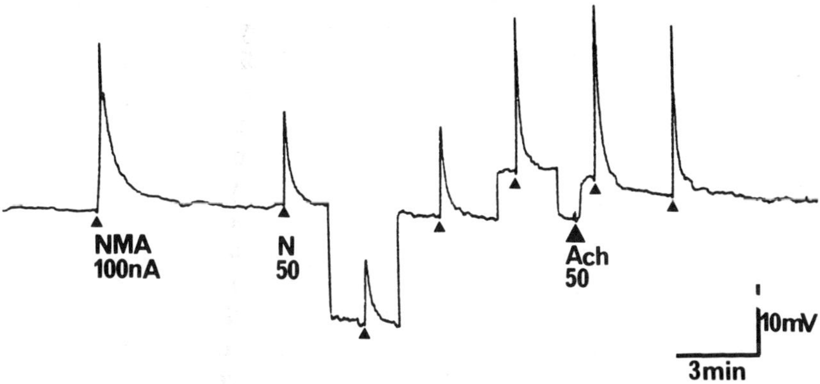

FIG. 7. Interactions between effects of NMDA and ACh, recorded intracellularly from a neuron in CA1. NMDA causes a large depolarization at 100 nA, and a smaller one at 50 nA. The response at 50 nA is voltage-dependent, as indicated by the reduction in amplitude when the neuron is hyperpolarized by passing current through the bridge circuit, and increased in amplitude when the cell is depolarized. When ACh is applied at resting potential (–55 mV), there is a depolarization to a value near to that previously applied by current. However, now the response to NMDA is larger than that recorded previously, even in the presence of the depolarizing current. The increase in response amplitude persists through the end of the trace, even though the level of depolarization has decayed. These observations indicate that the NMDA response is potentiated by action of ACh.

Because the M channel is the only channel affected in most of these neurons, there often is little or no effect of acetylcholine application onto neurons at resting potential. In fact, only about 13% of neurons onto which acetylcholine was applied were sufficiently excited to result in spike generation (ffrench-Mullen *et al.*, 1983). However, all neurons examined systematically showed the presence of M channels turned off by acetylcholine when tested by looking for interactions of acetylcholine with excitatory amino acids, or when recording intracellularly. Results from this type of study are shown in Figures 6 and 7. Figure 6 shows that if acetylcholine is ionophoresed prior to ionophoretic application of glutamate, the glutamatic response is increased when the potential is adjusted to be the same as the control. After ionophoretic application of acetylcholine, the response to a constant glutamate pulse was increased in both amplitude and duration. At a higher glutamate current this effect is less clear, but there is still an increase in response duration. In Figure 7, from a hippocampal neuron, the effect of acetylcholine application on the response to NMDA is shown. NMDA (N), when applied at 50 nA, gave a submaximal response, which is also voltage-dependent in the same range of membrane potential, but is due to a different mechanism from that of the M channel. The NMDA channel is blocked in its open configuration by Mg^{2+}, but this blockade is removed at more depolarizing potentials. Thus, the NMDA response is less at hyperpolarized potentials and greater at depolarized potentials than at resting potential. Thus, these observations suggest that acetylcholine is not a very effective transmitter for directly depolarizing the neuron, but has great ability to alter the effectiveness of other excitatory inputs which move membrane potential into the region of M channel activation.

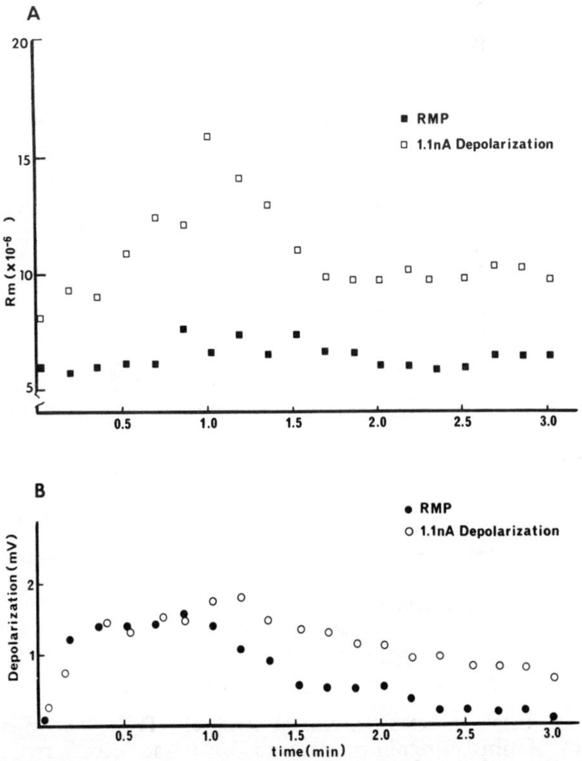

FIG. 8. Membrane resistance (Rm) and voltage changes induced by ionophoretic ACh in an experiment with intracellular recording of ACh responses of a neuron in rat piriform cortex. The neuron had a resting potential of –68 mV. (A) Resistance changes as a function of time after a 5-sec pulse of ACh (200 nA), applied first at resting membrane potential (closed symbols) and then in the presence of a constant depolarizing current of 1.1 nA (open symbols). The resistance was measured from the voltage shift produced by a 1 nA depolarizing pulse, 30 msec in duration. (B) Voltage shift produced by the same application as a function of time. (From ffrench-Mullen *et al.*, 1983; used with permission.)

Figure 8 is a plot of the changes in resistance and potential induced in a piriform cortex neuron upon ionophoretic application of acetylcholine. At resting potential (–68 mV in this neuron), there is only a small depolarization and almost no measurable change in input resistance. However, when the neuron was depolarized by application of a 1.1 nA current, the same acetylcholine application induced a clear and long-lasting increase in the membrane resistance, accompanied by a prolonged depolarization of the membrane potential. These results are consistent with the interpretation that upon depolarization the M channels in this neuron are opened, tending to restore potential toward control. Upon application of acetylcholine, the M channels are closed, resulting in an increase in resistance which can then result in an increased effectiveness of other depolarizing inputs.

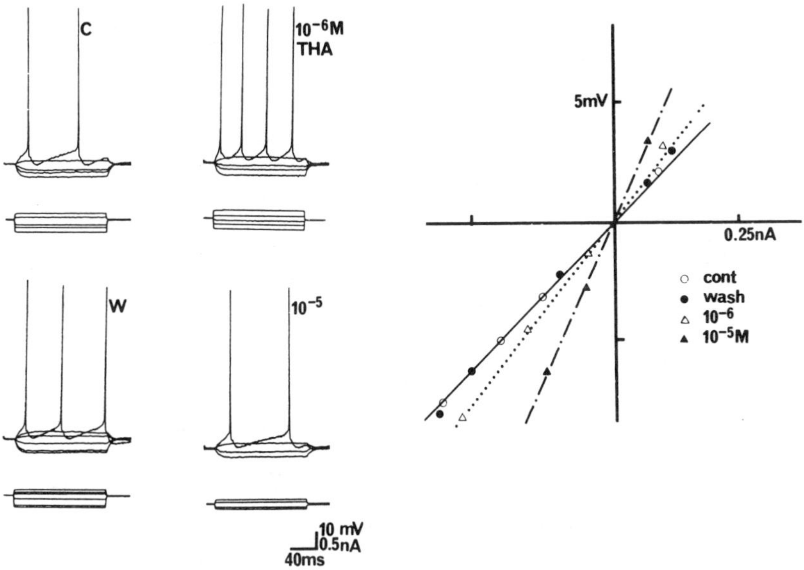

FIG. 9. Effects of tetrahydroaminoacridine (THA) on membrane properties of hippocampal neurons recorded intracellularly in CA1. The records on the left show the effects of passing pulses of depolarizing and hyperpolarizing current steps on membrane potential in the control (C), presence of 10^{-6}M THA, Wash (W) and presence of 10^{-5}M THA. The current-voltage relation obtained from such study is shown at the right. Note that there is a dose-dependent increase in input resistance in presence of THA, even when no ACh was applied. These results suggest that there is a background effect of endogenous ACh even in absence of exogenous application. Resting membrane potential was –55 mV, and the voltage excursions are too small for the voltage-dependence of the ACh response.

THA is an antiacetylcholinesterase that has been found to have some benefit in reducing the symptoms of Alzheimer's disease (Summers *et al.*, 1986). Figure 9 shows the results of application of THA onto a hippocampal slice, in which intracellular recordings were made and membrane resistance monitored. This figure shows a dose-dependent increase in membrane resistance induced by THA, which is similar to that induced by application of acetylcholine. The voltage-dependent nature of the resistance increase is less obvious in this particular neuron, probably because the resting potential was –57 mV. There was an increased tendency toward repetitive discharge in the presence of THA, similar to that caused by acetylcholine application.

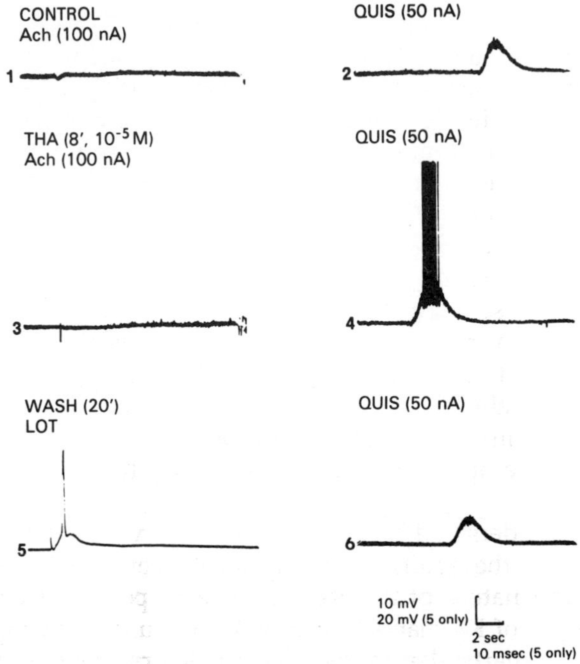

FIG. 10. Effects of THA on responses to ACh and quisqualate (QUIS) recorded intracellularly from a neuron in piriform cortex. Resting membrane potential of this neuron was −63 mV. Trace 1 shows that there is effectively no response to ACh at resting potential, while in trace 2, 50 nA of QUIS causes a depolarizing response. In presence of THA there is little or no increase in the ACH response, but the QUIS response is greatly increased, presumably as a result of the fact that the depolarization induced by QUIS moves the membrane potential into the range where ACh can block the M channels. The effect is reversible as shown in trace 6. Record % is a recording of the synaptic potential induced by stimulation of the lateral olfactory tract in this neuron. Note the action potential superimposed on the EPSP.

Figure 10 shows that THA alters the responses to ionophoretic application of excitatory amino acid agonists in a fashion similar to that of acetylcholine. In this experiment from a piriform cortex neuron, there was no obvious response to 100 nA acetylcholine either before or after perfusion of THA. However, the response to ionophoretic quisqualate, paired to and following the acetylcholine application, was dramatically increased in the presence of THA. The effect was reversible with washing. This result suggests that the therapeutic effect of THA is correlated with an increased efficacy of turning off M channels via a reduction in the breakdown of acetylcholine released from endogenous stores.

Discussion

The evidence for a particular role for acetylcholine in understanding neuronal deficits in aging comes from two primary sources. It has been known for a long time that muscarinic acetylcholine antagonists, such as scopolamine, have the effect of blocking short-term memory when given to normal individuals (Drachman and Leavitt, 1974). Since loss of short-term memory is a prime feature of various dementias, this fact suggests at least the possibility that muscarinic receptors play an important role in recall. In addition, there is good evidence that in Alzheimer's disease there is a dramatic loss of cholinergic innervation of the cortex, primarily as a result of loss of the neurons in the nucleus basalis of Meynert (Coyle *et al.*, 1983; Whitehouse *et al.*, 1981). While there is considerable debate as to whether or not the loss of these neurons is the cause of the disease (Maragos *et al.*, 1987), it is clear that at least some of the symptoms result from the loss of cholinergic innervation.

In order to understand how cholinergic innervation may play a role in memory and the ability to recall recent events, it is necessary to understand the nature of the acetylcholine response. M channels are one of a variety of K^+ channels, but they have unusual properties that make them of particular importance in determining excitability of neurons. Since M channels are opened whenever membrane potential moves into the depolarized zone of less than –60 mV, they have the effect of limiting the duration of any excitatory stimulus. Thus, when a synaptic input occurs, the membrane potential depolarizes and the neuron discharges. The depolarization, however, opens the M channels and tends to restore potential to resting levels via two mechanisms: the increased K^+ conductance tends to hyperpolarize the cell, and at the same time the decrease in the input resistance of the cell tends to reduce the excitatory drive caused by the synaptic input. Thus, the net result of M channels is to reduce repetitive discharge, and severely limit the duration of excitation.

The major role of acetylcholine in the central nervous system appears to be to turn off M channels, and by so doing, to increase electrical excitability and promote repetitive discharge. This is accomplished by the inverse of the mechanisms indicated above. There is a depolarization, albeit one that is relatively small and apparent in only some neurons. The more important feature is probably the increase in input resistance and the fact that the duration of the acetylcholine effect is prolonged. Thus, acetylcholine makes the neurons much more excitable to any depolarizing stimulus. In fact, by virtue of the increase in input resistance, acetylcholine will also make the neuron more sensitive to inhibitory inputs.

Acetylcholine is not the only transmitter known to be coupled to M channels, since luteinizing hormone release hormone (Brown and Adams, 1980) and angiotensin II (Brown *et al.*, 1980) have similar actions.

The mechanisms by which the nervous system stores information about past events is still very unclear, but the process of long-term potentiation provides at least one model of a process whereby events at a particular synapse may change in a long-term or even permanent fashion the excitability at that synapse. No one would propose that long-term potentiation is the only substrate of memory, but it probably is at least one important mechanism. Long-term potentiation is most prominent in those structures like hippocampus that are known to be very important sites for storage of short-term memory. It also occurs throughout the central nervous system but not to any great extent in the spinal cord or the peripheral nervous system (Teyler and DiScenna, 1987).

While the mechanism to LTP is also a subject of debate, and indeed there is a major controversy at present on whether LTP is primarily pre- or post-synaptic (Bekkers and Stevens, 1990; Malenka *et al.*, 1988), our results implicate acetylcholine receptors in the process, since it is prevented by scopolamine. Certainly it is not only muscarinic receptors that are important in LTP, as it is known that NMDA receptors play a particularly important role in some (Collingridge *et al.*, 1983) but not all (Harris and Cotman, 1986) sites. It seems likely that the role of muscarinic receptors may be related to factors discussed above; that is, without acetylcholine the M channels open to such a degree that the depolarization that triggers LTP is inadequate. Further investigations of this effect are merited, however.

Obviously, normal functioning of the brain requires the normal and integrated actions of a great variety of neurotransmitters, peptides and hormones. There is considerable redundancy in the central nervous system, and this takes the form of multiple transmitters being coupled to the same ionic mechanism, as is the case for M channels. Nonetheless, it is clear that muscarinic acetylcholine receptors are very important in this function.

Acknowledgements

This work was supported by NIH grant RO1 NS23807. We thank Mrs. Charlene McAuliffe for secretarial assistance.

References

Adams, R. R. and Brown, D. A. (1980). Luteinizing hormone-releasing factor and muscarinic agonists act on the same voltage-sensitive K^+ current in bullfrog sympathetic neurons. *Brit. J. Pharmacol.*, **68:** 353-355.

Adams, P. R., Brown, D. A. and Cionstanti, A. (1982). Pharmacologic inhibition of the M-current. *J. Physiol. (Lond.)*, **332:** 223-262.

Bartus, R. T., Beer, R. L. D. B. and Lippa, A. S. (1982). The cholinergic hypothesis of geriatric memory dysfunction. *Science*, **217:** 408-417.

Becker, R. E. and Giacobini, E. (1988). Mechanisms of cholinesterase inhibition in senile dementia of the Alzheimer type: Clinical, pharmacological, and therapeutic aspects. *Drug Dev. Res.*, **12:** 163-195.

Bekkers, J. M. and Stevens, C. F. (1990). Presynaptic mechanism for long-term potentiation in the hippocampus. *Nature*, **346:** 724-729.

Brinkman, S. D. and Gershon, S. (1983). Measurement of cholinergic drug effects on memory in Alzheimer's disease. *Neurobiol. Aging*, **4:** 139-145.

Brown, D. A. and Adams, P. R. (1980). Muscarinic suppression of a novel voltage-sensitive K^+ current in a vertebrate neurone. *Nature*, **283:** 673-676.

Brown, D. A., Constanti, A. and Marsh, S. (1980). Angiotensin mimics the action of muscarinic agonists on rat sympathetic neurones. *Brain Res.*, **193:** 614-619.

Christie, J. E., Shering, A., Ferguson, J. and Glen, A. I. M. (1981). Physostigmine and arecoline: Effects of intravenous infusions in Alzheimer presenile dementia. *Brit. J. Psychiat.*, **138:** 46-50.

Collingridge, G. L., Kehl, S. J. and McLennan, H. (1983). Excitatory amino acids in synaptic transmission in the Schaffer-commissural pathway of the rat hippocampus. *J. Physiol. (Lond.)*, **334:** 33-46.

Coyle, J. T., Price, D. L. and DeLong, M. (1983). Alzheimer's disease: A disorder of cortical cholinergic innervation. *Science*, **219:** 1184-1190.

Crystal, H., Dickson, D., Fuld, P., Masur, D., Scott, R., Mehler, M., Masdeu, J., Kawas, C., Aronson, M. and Wolfson, L. (1988). Clinico-pathologic studies in dementia: Nondemented subjects with pathologically confirmed Alzheimer's disease. *Neurology*, **38:** 1682-1687.

Davis, P. and Mahoney, A. J. F. (1976). Selective loss of central cholinergic neurons in Alzheimer's disease. *Lancet*, **2:** 1403.

Deutsch, J. A. (1971). The cholinergic synapse and the site of memory. *Science*, **174:** 788-794.

Drachman, D. A. and Leavitt, J. (1974). Human memory and the cholinergic system: A relationship to aging? *Arch. Neurol.*, **30:** 113-121.

Elrod, K. and Buccafusco, J. J. (1988). An evaluation of the mechanism of scopolamine-induced impairment in two passive avoidance protocols. *Pharmacol. Biochem. Behav.*, **29:** 15-21.

ffrench-Mullen, J. M. H., Hori, N., Nakanishi, H., Slater, N. T. and Carpenter, D. O. (1983). Asymmetric distribution of acetylcholine receptors and M channels on prepyriform neurons. *Cell. Molec. Neurobiol.*, **3:** 163-181.

Glick, S. D., Mittag, T. W. and Green, J. P. (1973). Central cholinergic correlates of impaired learning. *Neuropharmacology*, **12:** 291-296.

Harbaugh, R. E., Roberts, D. W., Coombs, D. W., Saunders, R. L. and Reeder, T. M. (1984). Preliminary report: Intracranial cholinergic drug infusion in patients with Alzheimer's disease. *Neurosurgery*, **15:** 514-518.

Harris, E. W. and Cotman, C. W. (1986). Long-term potentiation of guinea pig mossy fiber responses is not blocked by N-methyl-D-aspartate antagonists. *Neurosci. Lett.*, **70:** 132-137.

Hirotsu, I., Hori, N., Katsuda, N. and Ishihara, T. (1989). Effect of anticholinergic drug on long-term potentiation in rat hippocampal slices. *Brain Res.*, **482:** 194-197.

Hori, N., Akaike, N. and Carpenter, D. O. (1988). Piriform cortex brain slices: Techniques for isolation of synaptic inputs. *J. Neurosci. Meth.*, **25:** 197-208.

Kelly, J. S., Dodd, J. and Dingledine, R. (1979). Acetylcholine as an excitatory and inhibitory transmitter in the mammalian central nervous system. *Prog. Brain Res.*, **49:** 253-266.

Kopelman, M. D. (1986). The cholinergic neurotransmitter system in human memory and dementia: A review. *J. Exper. Psychol.*, **38A:** 535-573.

Krnjevic, K. and Phillis, J. W. (1963). Acetylcholine sensitive cells in the cerebral cortex. *J. Physiol. (Lond.)*, **166:** 296-327.

Kuba, K. and Kumamoto, E. (1990). Long-term potentiations in vertebrate synapses: A variety of cascades with common subprocesses. *Prog. Neurobiol.*, **34:** 197-269.

Malenka, R. C., Kauer, J. A., Zucker, R. S. and Nicoll, R. A. (1988). Postsynaptic calcium is sufficient for potentiation of hippocampal synaptic transmission. *Science*, **242:** 81-87.

Maragos, W. F., Greenamyre, J. T., Penney J. B. Jr., and Young, A. B. (1987). Glutamate dysfunction in Alzheimer's disease: An hypothesis. *TINS*, **10:** 65-68.

Nussinovitch, I. and Rahamimoff, R. (1988). Ionic basis of tetanic and post-tetanic potentiation at a mammalian neuromuscular junction. *J. Physiol. (Lond.)*, **396:** 435-455.

Palmer, A. M. and Gershon, S. (1990). Is the neuronal basis of Alzheimer's disease cholinergic or glutamatergic? *FASEB*, **4:** 2745-2752.

Peterson, R. C. (1977). Scopolamine induced learning failures in man. *Psychopharmacology*, **52:** 283-289.

Smith, G. (1988). Animal models of Alzheimer's disease: Experimental cholinergic denervation. *Brain Res. Rev.*, **13:** 103- 118.

Spehlmann, R. (1963). Acetylcholine and prostigmine electrophoresis at visual cortical neurons. *J. Neurophysiol.*, **26:** 127-139.

Summers, W. K., Majovski, L. V., Marsh, G. M., Tachiki, K. and Kling, A. (1986). Oral tetrahydroaminoacridine in long-term treatment of senile dementia, Alzheimer type. *N. Engl. J. Med.*, **315:** 1241-1245.

Teyler, T. J. and DiScenna, P. (1987). Long-term potentiation. *Ann. Rev. Neurosci.*, **10:** 131-161.

Whitehouse, P. J., Price, D. L., Clark, A. W., Coyle, J. T. and DeLong, M. R. (1981). Alzheimer disease: Evidence for selective loss of cholinergic neurons in the nucleus basalis. *Ann. Neurol.*, **10:** 122-126.

Wigstrom, H., Gustafsson, B. and Huang, Y.-Y. (1986). Mode of action of excitatory amino acid receptor antagonists on hippocampal long-lasting potentiation. *Neuroscience*, **17:** 1105-1115.

Alterations in Muscarinic Cholinergic Neurotransmission in Normal Aging and Alzheimer's Disease: Implications for Current Therapeutic Strategies for Treatment of Dementia

ESAM E. EL-FAKAHANY[1] and JAMES A. JOSEPH[2]

[1] *Division of Neuroscience Research in Psychiatry, University of Minnesota Medical School, Box 392, Mayo Memorial Building, Minneapolis, MN 55455, USA*
[2] *Molecular Physiology and Genetics Section, Gerontology Research Center/NIA, Baltimore, MD 21224, USA*

Keywords

Muscarinic receptors, Subtypes, Aging, Alzheimer's disease, Dementia, Animal models, Humans, Phosphoinositide hydrolysis, Adenylate cyclase, Electrophysiological responses, Acetylcholine synthesis, Acetylcholine release, Receptor plasticity.

Abbreviations

mAChR: Muscarinic acetylcholine receptor
PI: Phosphoinositides
IP3: Inositol-1,4,5-trisphosphate

Introduction

It is well known that central cholinergic systems (e.g., in the hippocampus and basal forebrain) play a major role in the process of memory through the activation of muscarinic receptors (Bartus *et al.*,

1982). Given the marked deterioration of cognitive function in normal aging, and more notably in Alzheimer's disease, there has been continued active research to elucidate the possible deficits in cholinergic neurotransmission in these two conditions. Moreover, there have been numerous studies of the efficacy of different approaches of enhancing cholinergic neurotransmission in the brain in alleviating memory deficits in the elderly and in Alzheimer's patients. However, previous work has indicated only minimal success in improving performance in tasks that assess memory in senescent animals or humans with pharmacological agents which enhance cholinergic functioning (Sherman *et al.*, 1988; Flood and Cherkin 1988; Bartus and Dean, 1988). Furthermore, attempts to restore cognitive performance through the administration of such agents (e.g., tacrine) in patients suffering from dementing disorders, such as Alzheimer's disease, have yielded variable outcomes, ranging from modest, temporary improvement to mixed results (Sherman *et al.*, 1988; Bartus, 1990). Conversely, these agents are efficacious in improving performance in memory tasks in young animals lesioned in specific brain regions (e.g., hippocampus, nucleus basalis of Meynert) that are affected in Alzheimer's disease (Haroutunian *et al.*, 1985; Murray and Fibiger, 1985, 1986).

Thus, it appears that efforts to enhance cholinergic functioning via agents which alter the activity of cholinergic neurons in target structures are effective in young organisms but not in normal senescent subjects or in humans suffering from Alzheimer's disease. While there is a host of factors that could be responsible for these age-related alterations in pharmacologic efficacy, including kinetic differences or the involvement of multiple transmitter systems, one could postulate that there may be specific age- or disease-induced changes in mAChR or in their signal transduction mechanisms that are responsible for these changes.

The aim of the present review is to elucidate the synaptic changes that take place in muscarinic functioning and to suggest possible mechanisms responsible for the loss of mAChR responsiveness in normal senescence and Alzheimer's disease.

Effects of aging and Alzheimer's disease on presynaptic cholinergic mechanisms

Reports of the effects of aging on brain acetylcholine synthesis in experimental animals have been controversial and demonstrated no changes (Meyer *et al.*, 1986) or a decrease (Gibson and Peterson, 1980), with no major effects on steady-state levels of acetylcholine (Decker,

1987). This is in spite of the relatively consistent findings of a decline in the high-affinity, sodium-dependent, choline uptake with aging in different brain regions (Gibson and Peterson, 1980; Strong *et al.*, 1986; Gilad *et al.*, 1987; also see Decker, 1987 for a comprehensive review). However, the controversy regarding the changes in acetylcholine synthesis might be related to the small effects, or no effects, of aging on the activity of choline acetyltransferase in different brain regions of humans and laboratory animals (reviewed in Decker, 1987). The reasons for these inconsistent findings are numerous and could include assay procedures (Waller *et al.*, 1983), or sex/strain/species differences (Luine *et al.*, 1986; Strong *et al.*, 1980). One other important consideration is the precise localization of the neural area utilized for the assay.

The results with respect to acetylcholinesterase have been even more controversial than those for other parameters. Various studies have indicated that declines range from 0 to 26% in aged rodents and are less than 20% in the aged human (Morin and Wasterlain, 1980). Thus, the variability of these results makes it difficult to explain aging-associated memory deficits according to significant changes in presynaptic cholinergic function. In general, the changes in areas such as the hippocampus and cortex that occur as a function of normal aging are less reliable than those seen in Alzheimer's disease, particularly with respect to the marked reduction in choline acetyltransferase activity in this disease (Coyle *et al.*, 1983).

Effects of aging and Alzheimer's disease on the concentration of muscarinic receptors in the brain

Several investigators have studied the effects of normal aging on the concentration of mAChR in various brain regions of experimental animals using radioligand binding techniques. A summary of the findings of such studies is presented in Table 1. In general, normal aging is associated with a statistically significant decrease in receptor density in the majority of brain regions, amounting to about 20-30%. Autoradiographic analysis revealed that the pattern of mAChR loss throughout the brain was highest in areas such as the striatum which contain high concentrations of cholinergic perikaryon (Biegon *et al.*, 1989; Blake *et al.*, 1990). Thus, a selective loss of cholinergic neurons could be a contributing factor to the decline in mAChR concentration. Anatomically, there appears to be a close relationship between the distribution of mAChR within the striatum and the dopamine (D_2 subtype) receptors, being highest in the rostral region and lowest in the caudal portion of the striatum. mAChRs are lost as a function of age primarily from the medial and caudal portions of the striatum (Strong *et al.*, 1982).

Recent molecular biological evidence has indicated that there are as many as five mAChR subtypes (m1-m5) as indicated by the diversity of their genes, and specific cDNA probes have been developed for each subtype (Bonner, 1989). Unfortunately, at present, pharmacologic agents which distinguish clearly among all of the five mAChR subtypes have not been developed. However, there have been some efforts to determine the age-related loss of the m1 mAChR since it has been proposed that this particular receptor subtype plays an important role in memory (Messer *et al.*, 1987). Radioligand binding studies in brain homogenates have indicated that the effects of aging on muscarinic receptors are not the result of a preferential decrease in the m1 receptor subtype, as defined by the high affinity binding of the selective antagonist pirenzepine (Norman *et al.*, 1986; Surichamorn *et al.*, 1988). On the other hand, autoradiographic studies revealed a small decline (10-20%) in the density of m1 receptors (defined by the binding of [^{3}H]quinuclidinyl benzilate in the presence of a low concentration of the agonist carbachol) in several brain regions of aged rats (Biegon *et al.*, 1988). These regions include the anterior and parietal cortex and the striatum. Even smaller changes were noted in the ventral limb of the diagonal band, the CA3 field of the hippocampus and some nuclei of the amygdala. These results are in contrast to a report that the binding of [^{3}H]pirenzepine is higher in the cerebral cortex of aged Wistar rats (Sirvio *et al.*, 1988). Moreover, there was a marked decrease (25-30%) in the concentration of m2 muscarinic receptors (defined by binding of [^{3}H]quinuclidinyl benzilate in the presence of a low concentration of pirenzepine) in the medial septum, diagonal band, locus ceruleus, pontine nuclei and layers V and VI of the cerebral cortex (Biegon *et al.*, 1988). It is interesting to note in this regard that a recent study using oligonucleotide DNA probes to assess mRNA coding for the m1, m3, and m4 mAChR subtypes with *in situ* hybridization has indicated no age-related decrements in any rat brain region examined (Blake *et al.*, 1990). These findings suggest that the observed age-related decrease in mAChR concentration is not the result of a transcription deficit. Thus, it appears that aging mainly affects the efficiency of translation of the receptor protein or its rate of degradation. Alternatively, some age-related posttranslational modification of the receptor protein might take place.

Table 1. Effects of Aging on the Concentration of Brain Muscarinic Receptors in Experimental Animals.

Brain Region	Species/Strain	Effects of Aging	References
CEREBRAL CORTEX	Wistar rats	Decrease	Popova, and Petkov,1989
		No change	Michalek *et al*, 1989 Sirvio *et al*., 1988
	Fischer 344 rats	Decrease	Michalek *et al*, 1989 Waller & London, 1989 Pedigo *et al*., 1984 Norman *et al*., 1986
	Wistar-Kyto rats	Decrease	Gilad *et al*., 1987
	Brown-Norway rats	No change	Gilad *et al*., 1987
	Lewis rats	Increase	Gilad *et al*., 1987
	CD rats	Decrease	Gurwitz *et al*., 1987
	NMRI mice	Decrease	Pilch and Muller, 1988
HIPPOCAMPUS	Wistar rats	Decrease	Popova & Petkov, 1989 Michalek *et al*., 1989
	Fischer 344 rats	Decrease	Michalek *et al*., 1989 Waller & London, 1989 Pedigo *et al*., 1984 Surichamorn *et al*., 1988 Lippa *et al*., 1985 Pintor *et al*., 1988
	Wistar-Kyoto rats	No change	Gilad *et al*., 1987
	Brown-Norway rats	No change	Gilad *et al*., 1987
	Lewis rats	No change	Gilad *et al*., 1987
	Sprague-Dawley rats	Decrease	Amenta *et al*., 1989
	CD rats	Decrease	Gurwitz *et al*., 1987
STRIATUM	Wistar rats	Decrease	Popova & Petkov, 1989 Michalek *et al*., 1989

Table 1 continued

	Fischer 344 rats	Decrease	Michalek *et al.*, 1989 Waller & London, 1989 Pedigo *et al.*, 1984 Pintor *et al.*, 1988
	CD rats	Decrease	Gurwitz *et al.*,1987
HYPOTHALAMUS	Wistar rats	Decrease	Popova & Petkov, 1989
	Fischer 344 rats	Decrease	Lippa *et al.*, 1985
CEREBELLUM	CD rats Fischer 344 rats	Increase No change	Gilad *et al.*, 1987 Surichamorn *et al.*, 1988

[a] A decrease was detected using [^{3}H]N-methylscopolamine, but not [^{3}H]quinuclidinyl benzilate as a ligand.
[b] A decrease of 25%, although not statistically significant.
[c] Observed only in male rats.

Several additional points should be elaborated upon regarding mAChR loss in senescence. ***First,*** the decrease in receptor concentration is observed whether the data are expressed relative to tissue weight or protein content (Pedigo *et al.*, 1984), suggesting that it is not due to general changes in protein synthesis which might accompany aging. ***Second,*** these changes in receptor density were not associated, in most cases, with changes in ligand affinity. ***Third,*** there is evidence for the dependence of the effects of aging on muscarinic receptor density on both strain and sex (Gilad *et al.*, 1987) (see Table 1). ***Fourth,*** most studies have reported no changes in muscarinic receptor agonist binding affinity to the high and low receptor conformations or the relative proportions of these affinity states (Michalek *et al.*, 1989; Waller and London, 1989; Briggs *et al.*, 1982). Lippa *et al.* (1985), however, demonstrated that the partial agonist oxotremorine binds to the receptor with multiple affinities only in aged rats.

With regard to the age-related declines in mAChR concentrations in humans, the results have been somewhat more variable, possibly resulting from the differences in postmortem delay and tissue preservation conditions. As examples, Nordberg and Winblad (1981) reported a decrease in the concentration of muscarinic receptors in the anterior part of the hippocampus with aging. Similar results were published by Rinne (1987). Interestingly, this decrease occurs as early as 30-50 years of age, with no further significant decline at older age (Rinne, 1987). Age-related decreases in receptor concentration were also demonstrated in human frontal cortex (Rinne, 1987; Parry *et al.*, 1981) and striatum (Rinne, 1987; Allen *et al.*, 1983). In contrast, Davies and Verth (1978) reported no changes in muscarinic receptors with aging in 19 regions of human brain. Further studies using a larger sample size will be necessary to determine the nature of these controversial findings.

Weinberger *et al.* (1990) have recently reported a decrease in the density of mAChR in the parietotemporal cortex in Alzheimer's disease patients using *in vivo* single photon emission computed tomography. This decrease was localized to areas where maximal declines in glucose utilization were observed, suggesting it might reflect regional atrophic changes. These findings confirm those obtained by *in vitro* binding studies in the frontal and temporal cortex where a 30% decrease in Alzheimer's brains was detected (Reinikainen *et al.*, 1987; but also see Kellar *et al.* (1987) where no changes were found). It has also been reported using the latter techniques that there is a significant decrease in mAChR in the hippocampus in Alzheimer's disease patients as compared to age-matched controls (Reinikainen *et al.*, 1987; Nordberg *et al.*, 1986). Autoradiographic studies have localized such a decrease to the CA1 region of the hippocampus (Probst *et al.*, 1988). Interestingly, the number of mAChR per each hippocampal pyramidal cell increases in Alzheimer's disease, suggesting up-regulation of receptors in the population of neurons remaining in this neurodegenerative disease. This supports the hypothesis of Nordberg *et al.*, (1983) that there is a compensatory increase in receptor density as a result of loss of the ascending cholinergic input to the hippocampus.

The effects of Alzheimer's disease on the relative distribution of mAChR subtypes in the brain remain unresolved. For example, Mash *et al.* (1985) have reported a significant selective decrease in m2 receptors in the cerebral cortex (defined as the high affinity binding sites for agonists). Similar results were obtained in the hippocampus (Smith *et al.*, 1987; Rinne *et al.*, 1989). However, there are also reports of no changes in this particular receptor subtype in both regions (Reinikainen *et al.*, 1987; Kellar *et al.*, 1987; Probst *et al.*, 1988). As has been seen in so many other instances when postmortem tissue is examined, there are numerous experimental factors (e.g., delay in obtaining tissue, differences in dissection techniques, etc.) that could account for these differential findings between the studies. More work is needed to reach more definitive conclusions.

Effects of aging on muscarinic receptor plasticity

Neurotransmitter receptors are subject to regulation by the state of receptor activation. Thus, prolonged receptor stimulation by agonists (both *in vivo* and *in vitro*) results in a decrease in receptor concentration and sensitivity, while chronic receptor blockade by antagonists *in vivo* induces receptor up-regulation and supersensitivity (reviewed in Nathanson, 1987; El-Fakahany and Cioffi, 1990). For example, it has been shown in numerous studies through the utilization of a variety of procedures (e.g., 6-hydroxydopamine lesions and chronic administration of antipsychotics, estrogen or prolactin that dopamine receptors can be up-regulated both in young and old animals (Joseph *et al.*, 1988; also see Joseph and Roth, 1988b for review). Interestingly, these alterations are accompanied by improvements in motor behavior on a variety of tasks (Joseph and Roth, 1988a).

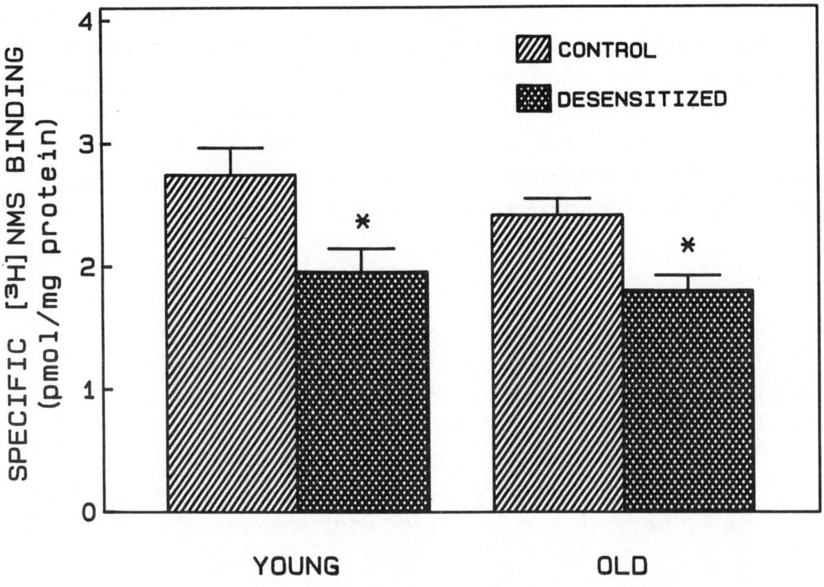

FIG. 1. Agonist-induced muscarinic receptor down-regulation in the cerebral cortex obtained from young (5-month-old) and old (22-24-month-old) Fischer 344 rats. Dissociated cells prepared from the cerebral cortex of both age groups were preincubated with (desensitized) or without (control) 1 mM oxotremorine-M for 3 hours at 37°C, followed by washing the agonist. Muscarinic receptors were then labeled with 2 nM [^{3}H]N-methylscopolamine ([^{3}H]NMS) for 1 hour at the same temperature. Nonspecific binding was measured in the presence of 2 μM atropine and was subtracted from total binding.
*Significantly lower than control within each age group, $P < 0.05$, but not different between the two ages. Reproduced from Surichamorn *et al.* (1989) with permission.

However, unlike the plasticity seen with respect to the dopamine receptors, the up-regulation of mAChR following their pharmacological blockade appears to be significantly impaired in aged rats and mice, at least in the cerebral cortex and hypothalamus (Pilch and Muller, 1988; Pedigo, 1988). These deficits are not seen with respect to mAChR down-regulation (Pintor *et al.*, 1988; Pilch and Muller, 1988) (Figure 1) and desensitization (Surichamorn, *et al.*, 1989) which occur to the same extent in young and aged rat brains. Further knowledge of the effects of aging on muscarinic receptor plasticity is of utmost importance, since cholinergic agonists and acetylcholinesterase inhibitors which are employed in treating memory deficits are usually used on a chronic basis. Moreover, centrally active drugs which belong to a variety of pharmacological classes attenuate mAChR activity (Pilch and Muller, 1988). These interactions result in troublesome side effects which usually become less manifest during prolonged treatment, possibly due to a compensatory supersensitivity of brain mAChR (Richelson and Nelson, 1984). Impairment of such receptor plasticity might result in persistence of these side effects in the elderly.

Impairment of signal transduction mechanisms associated with aging and Alzheimer's disease

As has been reviewed thus far, the alterations in presynaptic mechanisms (e.g., high affinity choline uptake, acetylcholinesterase activity, etc.) as a function of age appear to be variable and probably do not contribute significantly to the age-related memory deficits. Such presynaptic alterations, however, are thought to play an important role in the etiology of Alzheimer's dementia. Declines in mAChR concentration, as assessed with autoradiography and antagonist binding, appear to be at least partially responsible for memory loss and the observed decreased effectiveness of agents which enhance cholinergic neurotransmission in ameliorating memory deficits. This notion is supported by the absence of a significant population of spare receptors for a variety of mAChR-mediated signals in the brain (McKinney *et al.*, 1989) . However, although chronic treatment of either middle aged or aged animals with piracetam and dihydroergotoxine (hydergine) results in elevating the concentration of muscarinic receptors in the brain to the levels observed in young animals (Amenta *et al.*, 1989; Koide and Matsushita, 1981), these drugs alone appear to have very little effect on memory enhancement (see Bartus *et al.*, 1982).

The question therefore becomes, what other contributing mechanisms might be responsible for attenuating cholinergic function in aging and possibly in Alzheimer's disease? It has been suggested (Joseph and Roth, 1990; Joseph *et al.*, 1990) that decrements at any of several points in the signal transduction process following mAChR agonist interaction may contribute to the reduced agonist efficacy.

One of the most important signal transduction pathways coupled to the activation of mAChR in the brain is increased phosphoinositide (PI) hydrolysis, whereby the receptors mediate an increase in the breakdown of inositol-4,5-bisphosphate through the stimulation of phospholipase C (Fisher and Agranoff, 1987). This response involves coupling of muscarinic receptors to a guanine nucleotide binding protein (G-protein) (Litosch, 1987) and is triggered in mammalian brain by the activation of both m1 and m3 mAChR (Forray and El-Fakahany, 1990). One intracellular product resulting from this cleavage is inositol-1,4,5-trisphosphate (IP_3). Binding of IP_3 to specific receptors on the endoplasmic reticulum releases Ca^{2+} from storage sites within this cellular organelle and ultimately induces a physiological response (Fisher and Agranoff, 1987). Another important product of this signal transduction mechanism is the formation of diacylglycerol, which is an endogenous activator of protein kinase C (Nishizuka, 1984). It has been proposed that this particular protein kinase plays a vital role in learning and memory (Hu *et al.*, 1987).

Recent studies utilizing a variety of paradigms to assess loss of mAChR agonist responsiveness in senescence have indicated that the locus (i) of these deficits might be in the signal transduction pathways. For example, it has been shown that there is a decreased ability of muscarinic agonists to regulate striatal K^+-induced dopamine release through mAChR heteroreceptors (Joseph and Roth, 1988a; Joseph *et al.*, 1988b, 1990). When nicotine was utilized to increase dopamine release or if release was enhanced via antagonism of the dopamine D_2 receptors, no age-related differences were observed (Joseph and Roth, 1988a, 1988b). Thus, these deficits in mAChR responsiveness appear to be specific to the striatal muscarinic control of dopamine release. There is also a decrease in the function of presynaptic mAChR autoreceptors which regulate the release of acetylcholine during aging (Cansolo *et al.*, 1986).

Additional experiments have shown that the alterations in mAChR responsiveness may extend to other brain regions, such as the hippocampus. In this latter region, both extracellular (Lippa *et al.*, 1985) and intracellular (Segal, 1982) recording studies have revealed a highly selective reduction in the ability of iontophoretically applied acetylcholine to increase the excitability of hippocampal pyramidal cells. Moreover, Lippa *et al.* (1985) also suggested that this diminished responsiveness began at about 15-16 months of age, at which time reductions in the burst firing rate of these cells to applied acetylcholine were observed. Further reductions were reported in the senescent (24 months) group (Haigler *et al.*, 1985). Interestingly, aged rats show enhanced responsiveness to mAChR agonists on some parameters (e.g., hypothermia and antinociception) (Pedigo *et al.*, 1984).

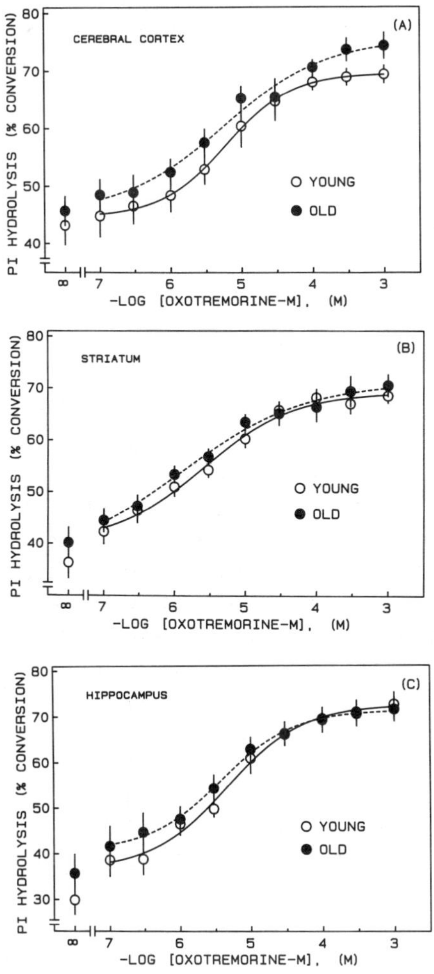

FIG. 2. Absence of effects of normal aging on muscarinic receptor-mediated phosphoinositide hydrolysis in various brain regions. Dissociated cell aggregates were prepared from the cerebral cortex (A), striatum (B) and hippocampus (C) of young (5-month-old) and old (22-24-month-old) Fischer 344 rats. Cells were labeled with [^{3}H]myo-inositol as described in Surichamorn *et al.* (1989). Phosphoinositide hydrolysis was induced by increasing concentrations of oxotremorine-M in the presence of 10 mM LiCl for 60 min at 37°C. The data are presented as a percentage conversion of inositol phospholipids into total inositol phosphates. Reproduced from Surichamorn *et al.* (1989) with permission.

Subsequent investigations carried out to assess the efficiency of signal transduction in the old rat have revealed putative deficits in this process. Initial studies suggested that there are no age-related effects on mAChR mediation of the increase in PI hydrolysis (as measured by the accumulation of total inositol phosphates in the presence of lithium) in various regions of rat brain (Fig. 2) (Surichamorn *et al.*, 1989; Crews *et al.*, 1986; but also see Nalepa *et al.*, 1989 where an increase in the magnitude of the response was observed in the cerebral cortex). It is worth noting that these studies did not specifically examine the accumulation of the putative second messenger, IP_3, and that the determination of total inositol phosphates was made only after a 60-min incubation. However, Joseph *et al.* (1990) have shown that early mAChR agonist enhancement of IP_3 formation in the presence of 30 mM KCl is reduced in striatal tissue obtained from 24-month-old Wistar rats. Moreover, it appears that there is not only diminished IP_3 accumulation but also a reduction of its efficacy to elicit Ca^{2+} mobilization from cortical microsomes of aged rats (Burnett *et al.*, 1990). This latter finding is interesting, since additional studies have indicated that there were no changes in either the density or affinity of IP_3 receptors in the cortex and cerebellum (W. S. Pou and E .E. El-Fakahany, unpublished observations) or in the striatum (Joseph and Roth, 1990; Joseph *et al.*, 1990). Moreover, a recent study has suggested that the age-related deficits in enhancement of K^+-evoked release of dopamine from striatal tissue could be reduced by "bypassing" the mAChR and mobilizing Ca^{2+} directly via the Ca^{2+} ionophore A23187 or by exogenous addition of IP_3 (Joseph *et al.*, 1988). These latter findings suggest that the age-related deficits in muscarinic signal transduction in the striatum may occur early in the process and may be due to a decrease in IP_3 formation as discussed above. In support of this hypothesis are recent findings from one of our laboratories (J. A. Joseph, unpublished data) which indicate: (1) no age-related differences in the ability of NaF, an activator of G-proteins to enhance K^+-evoked release of dopamine and IP_3 accumulation in the striatum; (2) reduced effectiveness of a GTP analog (GppNHp) to modulate the affinity of mAChR agonists. This latter finding indicates that the mAChR–G-protein complex is altered in senescence such that there is reduced coupling efficiency upon agonist stimulation.

In contrast, it has been shown that muscarinic receptor-mediated inhibition of adenylate cyclase activity in rat striatum and hippocampus (Rabin, 1986; Abdalah *et al.*, 1990) is not modified by normal aging. This response, at least in the striatum, is mediated by the activation of m4 muscarinic receptors (McKinney *et al.*, 1989) (using the nomenclature of Bonner, 1989).

In a recent review, it was suggested that signal transduction mechanisms also may be altered in Alzheimer's disease and that this may be responsible for the reduced efficacy of cholinergic replacement therapy (Fowler *et al.*, 1990). While there is still a paucity of research evidence and a great deal of variability in the postmortem samples examined, the research has suggested that Alzheimer's disease is accompanied by: (1) 40% reduction in the level of phosphatidylinositol concentration in the anterior temporal cortex (Stokes and Hawthorne, 1989); (2) 50% decrease in cytosolic protein kinase C levels in frontal cortex (Cole *et al.*, 1988); (3) 70% loss of IP_3 binding in temporal cortex and hippocampus (Young *et al.*, 1988); (4) attenuation of coupling of m1 mAChR to G-proteins in the cerebral cortex (Smith *et al.*, 1987; Flynn *et al.*, 1991).

Alternative approaches in treating memory deficits

As discussed above, cholinergic replacement therapy by a variety of procedures has been largely unsuccessful, or at least unreliable, in restoring memory function in senescence or in Alzheimer's disease. It is likely that this is in part due to subsensitivity of mAChR. Therefore, alternative approaches should be sought for alleviating memory deficits as a result of this disease.

Recent evidence from Dr. Joseph's laboratory (Joseph and Roth, 1990) has indicated that it is possible to "resensitize" the mAChR in striatal tissue from senescent animals by taking advantage of the "cross-talk" (Hill and Kendall, 1989) that exists between different second messenger systems. To elaborate, following mAChR stimulation by agonists, second messengers such as IP_3 must reach a certain threshold for a response to take place. Since this does not appear to occur in old animals, an alternative approach was tried to lower the second messenger threshold necessary for a response to be triggered by simultaneously activating and inhibiting more than one second messenger system. It is known that the mAChR agonist carbachol both stimulates PI hydrolysis and inhibits cyclic AMP formation in mammalian brain (Fisher and Agranoff, 1987; Forray and El-Fakahany, 1990; Anderson and McKinley, 1988). In contrast, oxotremorine primarily inhibits cyclic AMP levels and has little effect on PI hydrolysis (Anderson and McKinney, 1988). Joseph *et al.* (1991) determined the effects of combined application of carbachol and oxotremorine to perfused striatal slices from old animals on K^+-evoked dopamine release. As reported previously, Joseph and Roth, 1990), enhancement of K^+-evoked dopamine release was lower in striatal tissue from 24-month-old animals to either of these agents applied alone and that this was accompanied by reduced IP_3 formation (Table

2). However, simultaneous application of the two agonists enhanced K^+-evoked dopamine release to the same extent in the striatal tissue from young and old animals, even though age differences in IP_3 formation remained (Table 2) (Joseph *et al.*, in preparation). Moreover, co-application of arachidonic acid, which has a variety of direct and indirect second messenger effects (see Axelrod *et al.*, 1988 for review) with either carbachol or oxotremorine, also produced enhancement of K^+-evoked dopamine release to the same extent in striatal tissue from young and old animals (Table 2) (Joseph *et al.*, in preparation). Thus, these findings suggest that until research efforts determine the locus (or loci) of the age-related deficits in muscarinic function (i.e., G-protein coupling, alterations in receptor structure, etc.) methods to improve mAChR functioning might utilize procedures which can affect more than one second messenger system simultaneously. Synergistic activity among these systems may greatly facilitate neuronal transmission and subsequent physiological responses.

Table 2. Effects of Various Combinations of Carbachol, Oxotremorine and Arachidonic Acid on Dopamine and IP_3 Release in the Striata of Young and Aged rats

(PMOLES /mg PROTEIN; MEANS ± SEM)

	Dopamine release		**IP_3 release**	
	6 month	24 month	6 month	24 month
KCl	104 ± 7	104 ± 7	0	0
Carb.	155 ± 12	100 ± 8	80 ± 2	40 ± 3
Oxo.	161 ± 9	103 ± 10	32 ± 3	10 ± 2
Oxo.+ Carb.	163 ± 12	175 ± 15	30 ±1	50 ± 5
Arach.	158 ± 13	85 ± 10		
Arach.+ Oxo.	159 ± 11	160 ± 5		
Arach.+ Carb.	178 ± 4	157 ± 13		

KCl, 30 mM; Oxotremorine (Oxo.), 500 μM; Carbachol (Carb.), 500 μM; Arachidonic acid (Arach.), 10 μM

Alternatively, multiple neurotransmitter systems which are coupled to memory and cognition could be activated in concert, e.g., mAChR and glutamate receptors. Targeting IP_3 receptor-mediated regulation of intracellular Ca^{2+} signaling might also prove useful, e.g., by designing drugs which mimic the effects of IP_3. As mentioned above, however, the concentration of IP_3 receptors and the ability of IP_3 to mobilize intracellular Ca^{2+} are diminished in Alzheimer's disease and aging, respectively.

Conclusions

There is an extensive body of literature related to the effects of aging on muscarinic cholinergic neurotransmission in the central nervous system. However, careful review of such literature reveals that age-associated changes in the presynaptic components of this system in terms of acetylcholine synthesis are rather small, and in some cases controversial. It also becomes obvious that some of the detected changes are somewhat dependent on the animal species, strain and sex. Taken together, the "presynaptic" deficiencies in cholinergic neurotransmission which accompany normal aging cannot fully explain aging-associated memory deficits, in spite of the important role the cholinergic system plays in the process of memory. Some of these presynaptic deficits are more marked in Alzheimer's disease. However, it appears that the failure of cholinergic replacement therapy, both in normal aging and in Alzheimer's disease, may be the result of "postsynaptic" deficits in signal transduction as well as reduced mAChR concentration. Future research efforts should be focused upon reducing or reversing these signal transduction deficits in order to restore cholinergic functioning in these conditions. For example, research should concentrate on the following goals: (1) determination of the nature of reduced mAChR plasticity in senescence; (2) investigation of the mechanisms of reduced mAChR–G-protein coupling in senescence and Alzheimer's disease; (3) the design of agents which would cross-activate/inhibit more than one mAChR-linked second messenger system; (4) the design of therapeutic agents which could bypass mAChR and directly activate signal transduction pathways coupled to these receptors.

Acknowledgements

The authors would like to thank Ms. Donna Bethea for her secretarial help and Mr. Mike Gentry for his invaluable assistance. The work from the laboratory of E.E.E. was supported by grants AG-07118, NS-25743 and Research Career Development Award AG-00344 from the National Institutes of Health and by contract DAAL-03-88-0078 from the U.S. Army Research Office.

References

Abdalah, E. A. M., Pou, W. S. and El-Fakahany, E. E. (1990). Aging does not alter muscarinic receptor-mediated inhibition of cyclic AMP formation in the striatum and hippocampus. *Brain Res.* **534**: 234-236.

Allen, S. J., Benton, J. S., Goodhardt, M. D., Haan, E. A., Sims, N. R., Smith, C. C. T., Spillane, J. A., Bowen, D. M. and Davison, A. N. (1983). Biochemical evidence of selective nerve cell changes in the normal aging human and rat brain. *J. Neurochem.* **41**: 256-265.

Amenta, F., Cavallotti, C., Franch, F. and Ricci, A. (1989). Muscarinic cholinergic receptors in the hippocampus of the aged rat: effects of long-term hydergine administration. *Arch. Int. Pharmacodyn.* **297**: 225-234.

Anderson, D. J. and McKinney, M. (1988). Muscarinic M_2 receptor-mediated cyclic AMP reduction in mechanically dissociated rat cortex. *Brain Res.* **475**: 28-34.

Axelrod, J., Burch, R. M. and Jelsema, C. L. (1988). Receptor mediated activation of phospholipase A_2 via GTP-binding proteins: arachidonic acid and its metabolizers as second messengers. *Trends Neurosci.* **11**: 117-123.

Bartus, R. T. (1990). Drugs to treat age-related neurodegenerative problems. The final frontier of medical sciences. *J. Amer. Geriatrics Soc.* **38**: 680-695.

Bartus, R. T. and Dean, R. L. (1988). Tetrahydroaminoacridine, 3,4-diaminopyridine and physostigmine: direct comparison of effects on memory in aged primates. *Neurobiol. Aging* **9**: 351-356.

Bartus, R. T., Dean, R. L., Beer, B. and Lippa, A. S. (1982). The cholinergic hypothesis of geriatric memory dysfunction. *Science* **214**: 408-417.

Biegon, A., Duvdevani, R., Greenberger, V. and Segal, M. (1988). Aging and brain cholinergic muscarinic receptors: an autoradiographic study in the rat. *J. Neurochem.* **51**: 1381-1385.

Biegon, A., Hanau, M., Greenberger, V. and Segal, M. (1989). Aging and brain cholinergic muscarinic receptor subtypes: an autoradiographic study in the rat. *Neurobiol. Aging* **10**: 305-310.

Blake, M. D., Appel, N. M., Joseph, J. A., Stagg, C. A., Anson, M., De Souza, E. B. and Roth, G. S. (1990). Muscarinic acetylcholine receptor subtype mRNA expression and ligand binding in the aged rat brain. *Neurobiol. Aging.*

Bonner, T. I. (1989). The molecular basis of muscarinic receptor diversity. *Trends Pharmacol. Sci.* **12**: 148-151.

Briggs, R. S., Petersen, M. M. and Cook, P. J. (1982). Muscarinic agonist receptor subtypes in aging rat brain. *Neurobiol. Aging* **3**: 259-261.

Burnett, D. M., Daniell, L. C. and Zahniser, N. R. (1990). Decreased efficacy of inositol 1,4,5-trisphosphate to elicit calcium mobilization from cerebrocortical microsomes of aged rats. *Mol. Pharmacol.* **37**: 566-571.

Cansolo, S., Wang, J.-X., Fiorentini, F. and Vezzani, A. (1986). *In vivo* and *in vitro* studies on the regulation of cholinergic neurotransmission in striatum, hippocampus and cortex of aged rats. *Brain Res.* **374**: 212-218.

Cole, G., Dobkins, K. R., Hansen, L. A., Terry, R. D. and Saitoh, T. (1988). Decreased levels of protein kinase C in Alzheimer brain. *Brain Res.* **452**: 165-174.

Coyle, J. T., Price, D. L. and DeLong, M.R. (1983). Alzheimer's disease: a disorder of cortical cholinergic innervation. *Science* **219**: 1184-1190.

Crews, F. T., Gonzales, R. A., Polovcik, R., Phillips, M. L., Theiss, C. and Raizada, M. (1986). Changes in receptor stimulated phosphoinositide hydrolysis in brain during ethanol administration, aging and other pathological conditions. *Psychopharmacol. Bull.* **22**: 775-780.

Davies, P. and Verth, A. H. (1978). Regional distribution of muscarinic cholinergic receptor in normal and Alzheimer's type dementia brains. *Brain Res.* **138**: 385-392.

Decker, M. W. (1987). The effects of aging on hippocampal and cortical projections of the forebrain cholinergic system. *Brain Res. Rev.* **12**: 423-438.

El-Fakahany, E. E. and Cioffi, C. L. (1990). Molecular mechanisms of regulation of neuronal muscarinic receptor sensitivity. *Membrane Biochem.* **9**: 9-27.

Fisher, S. K. and Agranoff, B. W. (1987). Receptor activation and inositol lipid hydrolysis in neural tissues. *J. Neurochem.* **258**: 7358-7363.

Flood, J. F. and Cherkin, A. (1988). Effect of acute arecoline, tacrine and arecoline post-training administration on retention in old mice. *Neurobiol. Aging* **9**: 5-8.

Flynn, D. D., Weinstein, D. A. and Mash, D. C. (1991). Loss of high affinity agonist binding to M1 muscarinic receptors in Alzheimer's disease: Implications for the failure of cholinergic replacement therapy. *Annals Neurol.*

Forray, C. and El-Fakahany, E. E. (1990). On the involvement of multiple muscarinic receptor subtypes in the activation of phosphoinositide metabolism in rat cerebral cortex. *Mol. Pharmacol.* **37**: 893-902.

Fowler, C. J., O'Neill, Garlind, A. and Cowburn, R. F. (1990). Alzheimer's disease: is there a problem beyond recognitions? *Trends Pharmacol. Sci.* **11**: 103-104.

Gibson, G. E. and Peterson, C. (1980). Aging decreases oxidative metabolism and the release and synthesis of acetylcholine. *J. Neurochem.* **37**: 978-984.

Gilad, G. M., Rabey, J. M., Shenkman, L. and Gilad, V. H. (1987). Selective influence of rat genotype on age-related regional changes in forebrain muscarinic binding. *Neurobiol. Aging* **8**: 517-520.

Gurwitz, D., Egozi, Y., Henis, Y. I., Kloog, Y. and Sokolovsky, M. (1987). Agonist and antagonist binding to rat brain muscarinic receptors: influence of aging. *Neurobiol. Aging* **8**: 115-122.

Haigler, H. J., Cahill, L., Grager, M. and Charles, E. (1985). Acetycholine, aging and anatomy: differential effects in the hippocampus. *Brain Res.* **362**: 157-160.

Haroutunian, V., Kanof, P. and Davis, K. L. (1985). Pharmacological alleviation of cholinergic lesion-induced memory deficits in rats. *Life Sci.* **37**: 945-952.

Hill, S. J. and Kendall, D. A. (1989). Cross-talk between different receptor-effector systems in mammalian CNS. *Cell. Signal.* **1**: 135-141.

Hu, G. Y., Hvalby, O., Walaas, S. I., Albert, K. A., Skjeflo, P., Andrson, P. and Greengard, P. (1987). Protein kinase C injection into hippocampal pyramidal cells elicits features of long term potentiation. *Nature* **328**: 426-429.

Joseph, J. A. and Roth, G. S. (1988). Altered striatal dopaminergic and cholinergic reciprocal inhibitory control and motor behavioral decrements in senescence. In: *Proceedings of the First International Conference on Neuroimmunomodulation*, ed. W. Pierpaoli. *Ann. NY Acad. Sci.* **521**: 110-122.

Joseph, J. A. and Roth, G. S. (1988). Upregulation of striatal dopamine receptors and improvement of motor performance in senescence. In: *Central Determinants of Age Related Declines in Motor Function*, ed. J. A. Joseph. *Ann. NY Acad. Sci.* **515**: 355-366.

Joseph, J. A. and Roth, G. S. (1991). Loss of agonist receptor efficacy in senescence: Possible decrements in second messenger function and calcium mobilization. In: *Sandoz Lectures in Gerontology*, ed. C. Jesse. In press.

Joseph, J. A., Dalton, T. K. and Hunt, W. A. (1988). Age-related decrements in the muscarinic enhancement of K^+-evoked release of endogenous striatal dopamine: An indicator of altered cholinergic-dopaminergic reciprocal inhibitory control in senescence. *Brain Res.* **454**: 140-148.

Joseph, J. A., Dalton, T. K., Roth, G. S. and Hunt, W. A. (1988). Alterations in muscarinic control of striatal dopamine autoreceptors in senescence: a deficit at the ligand-muscarinic receptor interface? *Brain Res.* **454**: 149-155.

Joseph, J. A., Kowatch, M. D., Maki, T. and Roth, G. S. (1991). Selective cross activation/inhibition of second messenger systems and the reduction of age-related deficits in the muscarinic control of dopamine release from perfused rat striata. *Brain Res.*

Kellar, K. J., Whitehouse, P. J., Martino-Barrows, A. M., Marcus, K. and Price, D. L. (1987). Muscarinic and nicotinic cholinergic binding sites in Alzheimer's disease cerebral cortex. *Brain Res.* **436**: 62-68.

Koide, T. and Matsushita, H. (1981). An enhanced sensitivity of muscarinic cholinergic receptor associated with dopaminergic receptor subsensitivity after chronic antidepressant treatment. *Life Sci.* **28**: 1139-1145.

Lippa, A. S., Loullis, C. C., Rotrosen, J., Cardasco, D. M., Critchett, D. J. and Joseph, J. A. (1985). Conformational changes in muscarinic receptors may produce diminished cholinergic neurotransmission and memory deficits in aged rats. *Neurobiol. Aging* **6**: 317-323.

Litosch, I. (1987). Guanine nucleotide and NaF stimulation of phospholipase C activity in rat cerebral-cortical membranes. *Biochem. J.* 35-40.

Luine, V. N., Renner, K. J., Heady, S. and Jones, K. L. (1986). Age and sex-dependent decreases in ChAt in basal forebrain nuclei. *Neurobiol Aging* **7**: 193-198.

Mash, D. C., Flynn, D. D. and Potter, L. T. (1985). Loss of M2 muscarine receptors in the cerebral cortex in Alzheimer's disease and experimental cholinergic enervation. *Science* **228**: 1115-1117.

McKinney, M., Anderson, D. and Vella-Rountree, L. (1989). Different agonist-receptor active conformations for rat brain M_1 and M_2 muscarinic receptors that are separately coupled to two biochemical effector systems. *Mol. Pharmacol.* **35**: 39-47.

McKinney, M., Anderson, D., Forray, C. and El-Fakahany, E. E. (1989). Characterization of the striatal M2 muscarinic receptor mediating inhibition of cyclic AMP using selective antagonists: a comparison with the brainstem M2 receptor. *J. Pharmacol. Exp. Ther.* **250**: 565-572.

Messer, W. S., Thomas, G. J. and Hoss, W. (1987). Selectivity of pirenzepine in the central nervous system. II. Differential effects of pirenzepine and scopolamine on performance of a representational memory task. *Brain Res.* **407**: 37-45.

Meyer, E. M., Crews, F. T., Otero, D. H. and Larsen, K. (1986). Aging decreases the sensitivity of rat cortical synaptosomes to calcium ionophore-induced acetylcholine release. *J. Neurochem.* **47**: 1244-1246.

Michalek, H., Fortuna, S. and Pintor, A. (1989). Age-related differences in brain choline acetyltransferase, cholinesterases and muscarinic receptor sites in two strains of rats. *Neurobiol. Aging* **10**: 143-148.

Morin, A. M. and Wasterlain, C. G. (1980). Aging and rat brain muscarinic receptors as measured by quinuclidinyl benzilate binding. *Neurochem. Res.* **5**: 301-308.

Murray, C. L. and Fibiger, H. C. (1985). Learning and memory deficits after lesions of the nucleus basalis magnocellularis: reversed by physostigmine. *Neuroscience* **14**: 1026-1032.

Murray, C. L. and Fibiger, H. C., (1986). Pilocarpine and physostigmine attenuate spatial memory impairments produced by lesions of the nucleus basalis magnocellularis. *Behav. Neurosci.* **100**: 23-32.

Nalepa, S., Pinto, A., Fortuna, S., Vetulani, J. and Michalek, H. (1989). Increased responsiveness of the cerebral cortical phosphatidylinositol system to noradrenaline and carbachol in senescent rats. *Neurosci. Lett.* **10**: 195-199.

Nathanson, N. M. (1987). Molecular properties of the muscarinic acetylcholine receptor. *Ann. Rev. Neurosci.* **10**: 195-236.

Nishizuka, Y. (1984). The role of protein kinase C in cell surface signal transduction and tumor promotion. *Nature* **308**: 693-698.

Nordberg, A. and Winblad, B. (1981). Cholinergic receptors in human hippocampus: regional distribution and variance with age. *Life Sci.* **29**: 1937-1944.

Nordberg, A., Alafuzoff, I. and Winblad, B. (1986). Muscarinic receptor subtypes in hippocampus in Alzheimer's disease and mixed dementia type. *Neurosci. Lett.* **70**: 160-164.

Nordberg, A., Larsson, C., Adolfsson, R., Alafuzoff, I., and Winblad, B. (1983). Muscarinic receptor compensation in hippocampus of Alzheimer's patients. *J. Neural Transm.* **56**: 13-19.

Norman, A. B., Blaker, S. N., Thal, L. and Creese, L. (1986). Effects of aging and cholinergic deafferentation on putative muscarinic cholinergic receptor subtypes in rat cerebral cortex. *Neurosci. Lett.* **70**: 289-294.

Pedigo, N. W. (1988). Pharmacological adaptations and muscarinic receptor plasticity in hypothalamus of senescent rats treated chronically with cholineric drugs. *Psychopharmacol.* **95**: 497-501.

Pedigo, N. W. and Polk, D. M. (1985). Reduced muscarinic receptor plasticity in frontal cortex of aged rats after chronic administration of cholinergic drugs. *Life Sci.* **37**: 1443-1449.

Pedigo, N. W., Minor, L. D. and Krumrei, T. N. (1984). Cholinergic drug effects and brain muscarinic receptor binding in aged rats. *Neurobiol. Aging* **5**: 227-233.

Perry, E. K., Blessed, G., Tomlinson, B. E., Perry, R. N., Crow, T. J., Cross, A. J., Dockray, G. J., Dimaline, R. and Arregui, A. (1981). Neurochemical activities in human temporal lobe related to aging and Alzheimer type changes. *Neurobiol. Aging* **2**: 251-256.

Pilch, H. and Muller, W. E. (1988). Piracetam elevates muscarinic cholinergic receptor density in the frontal cortex of aged but not of young mice. *Psychopharmacol.* **94**: 74-78.

Pilch, H. and Muller, W.E. (1988). Chronic treatment with choline or scopolamine indicates the presence of muscarinic cholinergic receptor plasticity in the frontal cortex of young but not of aged mice. *J. Neural Transm.* **71**: 39-43.

Pintor, A., Fortuna, S., Volpe, M. T. and Michalek, H. (1988). Muscarinic receptor plasticity in the brain of senescent rats: down-regulation after repeated administration of diisopropyl fluorophosphate. *Life Sci.* **42**: 2113-2121.

Popova, J. S. and Petkov, M. D. (1989). Age-related changes in rat brain muscarinic receptors and β-adrenoreceptors. *Gen. Pharmacol.* **20**: 581-584.

Probst, A., Cortes, R., Ulrich, J. and Palacios, J. M. (1988). Differential modification of muscarinic. cholinergic receptors in the hippocampus of patients with Alzheimer's disease: an autoradiographic study. *Brain Res.* **450**: 190-201.

Rabin, R. A. (1986). Senescence does not alter activation or inhibition of striatal adenylate cyclase. *Neurobiol. Aging* **7**: 49-51.

Reinikainen, K. J., Reikkinen, P. J., Halonen, T. and Laakso, M. (1987). Decreased muscarinic receptor binding in cerebral cortex and hippocampus in Alzheimer's disease. *Life Sci.* 41: 453-461.

Richelson, E. and Nelson, A. (1984). Antagonism by antidepressants of neurotransmitter receptors of normal human brain *in vitro. J. Pharmacol. Exp. Ther.* **230**: 94-102.

Rinne, J. O. (1987). Muscarinic and dopaminergic receptors in the aging human brain. *Brain Res.* **40**: 162-168.

Rinne, J. O., Lonnberg, P., Marjamaki, P. and Rinne, U. K. (1989). Brain muscarinic receptor subtypes are differently affected in Alzheimer's disease and Parkinson's disease. *Brain Res.* **483**: 402-406.

Segal, M. (1982). Changes in neurotransmitter actions in the aged rat hippocampus. *Neurobiol. Aging* **2**: 99-104.

Sherman, K. A., Kumar, V., Ashford, J. W., Murphy, J. W., Eible, R. J. and Giacobini, E. (1988). Effect of oral physostigmine in senile dementia patients: Utility of blood cholinesterase inhibition and neuroendocrine response to define pharmacokinetics and pharmacodynamics. In: *Central Nervous System Disorders of Aging: Clinical Intervention and Research*, eds., R. Strong, W. G. Wood and W. J. Burke, Raven Press, New York, pp. 71-90.

Sirvio, J., Valjakka, A., Jolkkonen, J., Hervonen, A., and Riekkinen, P. J. (1988). Cholinergic enzyme activities and muscarinic binding in the cerebral cortex of rats of different age and sex. *Comp. Biochem. Physiol.* **90C**: 245-248.

Smith, C. J., Perry, E. K., Perry, R. H., Fairbairn, A. F. and Birdsall, N. J. M (1987). Guanine nucleotide modulation of muscarinic cholinergic receptor binding in postmortem human brain – a preliminary study in Alkheimer's disease. *Neurosci. Lett.* **82**: 227-232.

Stokes, C. E. and Hawthorne, J. N (1989). Reduced phosphoinositide concentration in anterior termporal cortex of Alzheimer-diseased brains. *J. Neurochem.* **48**: 1018-1021.

Strong, R., Hicks, P., Hsu, L., Bartus, R. T. and Enna, S. J. (1980). Age-related changes in the rodent brain cholinergic system and behavior. *Neurobiol. Aging* **1**: 59-63.

Strong, R., Rehwaldt, C. and Wood, W. G. (1986). Intra-regional variations in the effect of aging on high affinity choline uptake, choline acetyltransferase and muscarinic cholinergic receptors in rat neostriatum. *Exp. Gerontol.* **21**: 177-186.

Strong, R., Samorjski, T. and Gottesfeld, Z. (1982). Regional mapping of neostriatal neurotransmitter systems as a function of aging. *J. Neurochem.* **39**: 831-836.

Surichamorn, W., Abdallah, E. A. M. and El-Fakahany, E. E. (1989). Aging does not alter brain muscarinic receptor-mediated phosphoinositide hydrolysis and its inhibition by phorbol esters, tetrodotoxin and receptor desensitization. *J. Pharmacol. Exp. Ther.* **251**: 543-549.

Surichamorn, W., Kim, O. N., Lee, N. H., Lai, W. S. and El-Fakahany, E. E. (1988). Effects of aging on the interaction of quinuclidinyl benzilate, N-methylscopolamine, pirenzepine, and gallamine with brain muscarinic receptors. *Neurochem. Res.* **13**: 1183-1191.

Waller, S. B. and London, E. D. (1989). Choline acetyltransferase activity and muscarinic binding in brain regions of aging Fischer-344 rats. *Neurochem. Int.* **14**: 483-490.

Waller, S. B., Ingram, D. K., Reynolds, M. A. and London, E. D. (1983). Age and strain comparisons of neurotransmitter synthetic enzyme activities in the mouse. *J. Neurochem.* **41**: 1421 -1428.

Weinberger, D. R., Mann, U., Gibson, R. E., Coppola, R., Jones, D. W., Braun, A. R., Berman, K. F., Sunderland, T., Reba, R. C. and Chase, T. N. (1990). Cerebral muscarinic reecptors in primary degenerative dementia as evaluated by SPECT with iodine-123-labeled QNB. In: *Advances in Neurology, Vol. 51, Alzheimer's Disease,* eds., R. J. Wurtman *et al.*, Raven Press, New York, pp. 147-150.

Young, L. T., Kish, S. J., Li, P. P. and Warsh, J. J. (1988). Decreased brain [^{3}Hlinositol-1,4,5-trisphosphate binding in Alzheimer's disease. *Neurosci. Lett.* **94**: 198-202.

Influence of Normal Aging on Monoamines, Monoamine Receptors and Associated Signal Transduction Systems

MAYNARD H. MAKMAN

Departments of Biochemistry and Molecular Pharmacology, Albert Einstein College of Medicine, 1300 Morris Park Avenue, Bronx, New York 10461, U.S.A.

Introduction; general considerations

This chapter will consider various aspects of the influence of normal aging on the biochemistry of brain monoaminergic neurotransmitter systems, with a particular emphasis on the dopaminergic system. Also, for comparative purposes, there will be some discussion of age-related changes of the noradrenergic system in the myocardium. There has been at least some debate about the existence or the functional significance of nearly every putative age-associated change in the brain of normal human or normal experimental animal subjects. Included here is the extent and significance of neuronal loss with age. Thus, it is not surprising that there is controversy concerning what are the more significant age-related changes, and in particular what are the underlying mechanisms for those changes, in monoaminergic systems. Nevertheless, for monoaminergic systems a number of age-related changes have been reasonably well documented. In particular, dopaminergic and possibly also cholinergic systems may be the most sensitive to changes with age, although other transmitter systems also may be involved. Since all systems are not equally affected, as a consequence there is likely to be a change in balance. Many of the changes that occur during normal aging exhibit regional specificity and/or selectivity for neuronal cell type. This selectivity in fact argues against an "overall" nonselective effect of aging. It is often difficult to distinguish between primary and secondary or more complex indirect effects of aging. Neuroendocrine changes and peripheral changes may lead to changes in the central nervous system (CNS). Alternatively, CNS changes may be primary and lead to physiological aging.

It is also important to be aware of species differences and of strain differences within a given species for age-related changes. Thus there may be genetic factors operative within a given species, with differences found for different strains of mice and rats. Also there are differences in life span and in changes in body weight with age in different strains. As reviewed by Walford (1990), the H-2 major histocompatibility complex in mice, with certain H-2 antigens specifically or particularly involved, may play an important role (or provide important correlations at least) in age-associated events, possibly influencing diverse aspects, including receptor-signal transduction, superoxide dismutase and repair of oxidative damage, and reproductive senescence. Thus, certain specific strains of H-2 female congenic mice had the longest life span and also were able to bear litters later in life than other strains.

Dietary factors and environmental factors are often not given adequate consideration in aging studies. Alterations in the aged female animal depends on the animal's present reproductive status as well as on prior reproductive history (Weiland *et al.*, 1989). There is often a need for multiple time points in aging study to really have accurate information about whether a change occurs in "midlife" or with senescence. Also, changes in "midlife" may then be interactive with additional changes that occur later (e.g., possibly the case for dopamine D_1 and D_2 receptor interactions). In fact, it is not always clear at what age related changes are important. Some changes may not become of functional significance unless there is superimposed disease or stress. Finally, while it is important to investigate changes in very old animals, there is the added risk with such animals that (unknown) pathology may influence indirectly if not directly the parameters being investigated.

Age-related changes in monoamine systems in mammalian brain

Age-related loss of motor control, increased sensitivity to antidopaminergic drugs (dopamine D_2 receptor antagonists such as haloperidol), and the progressive nature of Parkinson's disease have been thought to be related to age-associated decreased functioning of the striatal (caudate/putamen) and possibly also other dopaminergic systems. These age-associated changes at least in part may be due to changes in dopamine receptors and/or in the functional coupling of dopamine receptors. In addition, there appear to be significant presynaptic changes. Certain changes may be species-specific. It appears from these changes that the nigrostriatal and possibly certain other dopaminergic systems are particularly sensitive to the aging process. Little is known to what extent this sensitivity is intrinsic to the organism, or to what extent environmental factors play a role. Overall, little is known about the molecular mechanisms involved. However, the biochemical changes in a number of instances correlate with and may account for behavioral changes (Randall *et al.*, 1981; Roth and Josephs, 1988). The reader is referred also to several reviews of this topic (Roth and Josephs, 1988; Morgan and Finch, 1988; Morgan and May, 1990; Horvath and Davis, 1990; Amenta *et al.*, 1991).

Monoamine concentration, synthesis, release and turnover

The number of monoamine-containing neurons show age-related decreases which appear to be specific for certain neuronal groups. Thus, not all monoamine systems "age" at the same rate (Weiland *et al.*, 1989; Tatton *et al.*, 1991). These decreases may occur in many instances without alteration in the number of terminals or in the concentration of amines in the terminals or tissue. Still, functional status may be altered and/or functional reserve may be diminished. Monoamine turnover may be increased as part of the compensation. Presynaptic changes may lead to postsynaptic changes, thereby modifying intrinsic age-related postsynaptic alterations, e.g., modifying age-related changes in postsynaptic receptor systems (see below). Turnover of monoamines in many cases is enhanced, probably in compensation for loss of transmitter (Carlsson, 1987).

Dopamine concentration, synthesis, release and turnover

It has been documented in a number of instances that the number of dopamine-containing neurons decreases with aging, yet tyrosine hydroxylase, the number of dopamine terminals and the concentration of dopamine may not be altered. Bowen (1984) found no change in tyrosine hydroxylase of human caudate during aging (from 50 to 100 years). Wolf *et al.* (1991) have studied as a function of aging synaptosomes from human caudate nucleus. Based on this study, the tyrosine hydroxylase protein content and the relative number of dopamine nerve terminals (synaptosomes) did not change as a function of age up to age 65. These investigators postulated therefore that there must have occurred a compensation for the previously documented loss of dopaminergic cell bodies with age. Kish *et al.* (1992) did find a progressive loss from 22 years to 84 years of age of dopamine content, together with an increased ratio of homovanillic acid (HVA) to dopamine, in human caudate nucleus and putamen. Kish and coworkers also reported that the regional and subregional patterns of loss of dopamine were different in normal aging and in Parkinson's disease; hence they postulated that the etiologies must be different. Although there is some conflicting data, dopamine content does not appear to be selectively decreased in Alzheimer's disease.

Osterburg *et al.* (1981) found no change in dopamine levels or turnover with aging in brain regions of male C57BL/6J mice from 4 months to 8-12 months of age, about a 20% decrease in dihydroxyphenylacetic acid (DOPAC) levels in striatum at 28 months, as well as some small changes in dopamine levels and turnover in median eminence-arcuate nucleus region of the older animals. There was a trend for decreased dopamine levels and turnover in hypothalamus after 34 months of age. Striatal dopamine concentration in the 24- and 28-month groups appeared to be about 30% lower than in the young animals. However, whether or not this was a consistent decrease was not clear, since levels appeared to be entirely normal at 21 and at 30 months. The authors mentioned that total striatal dopamine may be lower in the older animals, since striatal volume appears to be somewhat decreased.

We reported that striatal levels of dopamine were about 26% lower in 26-month than in 6-month-old Fischer 344 rats (Hirschhorn *et al.*, 1982). Also, we found in a comparison of 12- and 24-month-old rats, that stimulation of dopamine synthesis from tyrosine by forskolin was not at all impaired in striatal or hypothalamic synaptosomes from the old rats (Makman *et al.*, 1984). We have demonstrated that forskolin, an activator of adenylate cyclase, stimulates dopamine formation in dopaminergic synaptosomes *via* a cyclic AMP-dependent process (Katz *et al.*, 1983; Garber and Makman, 1987).

Marshall and Rosenstein (1990) have also carried out studies of age-related changes in striatal dopamine metabolism of Fischer 344 rats. The aged rats had less dopamine (about 20-35% less) as well as less dopamine metabolites (HVA and DOPAC) in striatal samples. The age-related decrease in dopamine appeared to occur uniformly throughout the striatum. Also, accumulation of dihydroxyphenylalanine (DOPA), following administration of the aromatic amino acid decarboxylase inhibitor NSD-1015, was decreased in the senescent animals. The decreases in dopamine content were evident late in the life span but not evident at 12 months of age (midlife).

Fernandez-Ruiz *et al.* (1992) reported sex differences in age-related changes in the dopaminergic system, with comparisons of 2-month and 24-26-month-old rats (female rats were in estrus). An age-related decrease in tyrosine hydroxylase in striatum of both sexes was found, with a more marked decrease in males; in limbic forebrain, tyrosine hydroxylase decreased only in males; and no significant age-related changes in tyrosine hydroxylase was found in hypothalamus of either sex. Dopamine content showed a decrease with age in female striatum (the only age-related change found). The dihydroxyphenylacetic acid (DOPAC): dopamine ratio (index of dopamine turnover) showed an age-related increase for all three regions in females; no significant change in any region in males. Gozlan *et al.* (1990) reported an age-associated decrease in dopamine content as well as an increased DOPAC:dopamine ratio. Rossi *et al.* (1992) found no age-associated change in tuberoinfundibular dopaminergic neurons of adenoma-free female rats with respect to tyrosine hydroxylase immunoreactivity or in number of dopaminergic neurons, while confirming the previously documented lactotroph hypertrophy and hyperplasia.

In a careful and significant study, Tatton *et al.* (1991) examined four monoaminergic neuronal populations in C57BL mice from 8 to 104 weeks of age with respect to possible age-related changes. The rates of neuronal loss for each group in which loss occurred could be expressed by a single exponential constant for the period of lifespan studied. Findings for locus coeruleus noradrenergic neurons and raphe serotonergic neurons are discussed later in this chapter. Two dopaminergic neuronal populations, substantia nigra dopaminergic neurons and retinal dopaminergic amacrine cells, were studied. There occurred a major loss of substantia nigra dopaminergic neurons, with an overall decline by the 104th week to only 30% of the neuronal number at 4 weeks still present. In marked contrast, there was essentially no loss of retinal dopaminergic neurons. Since other studies had indicated that there is little or no age-related change in striatal dopamine in this strain of mice (see also above), the authors conclude that striatal dopamine levels are maintained by a progressively smaller number of substantia nigra neurons with aging. In a companion study (Greenwood *et al.*, 1991) these investigators provided some evidence that the average surviving tyrosine hydroxylase and nigral neuron compensates for the age-related loss of other nigral neurons by increasing dopamine synthesis. This compensation may be mediated in part by increased synthesis of tyrosine hydroxylase. It was also noted that younger substantia nigra neurons that have survived low levels of toxically-induced damage (caused by 1-methyl-4-phenyl-1,2,3,6-tetrahydropyridine (MPTP)) behave in a similar fashion, i.e., compensate by increasing dopamine synthesis.

Of particular interest is a recent report of an age-dependent decrease in K^+-evoked dopamine release *in vivo* from striatum in the Fischer 344 rat (Friedmann and Gerhardt, 1992). Ventral striatum showed greater age-related decrements than did dorsal striatum. This study provides direct evidence for impaired presynaptic dopaminergic functional potential. Also in the same study differential effects of nomifensine suggested alteration of the dopamine uptake process as well. An age-related loss of K^+-stimulated dopamine release from striatal slices of male rats *in vitro* has also been reported (Dluzen *et al.*, 1988; Laping *et al.*, 1990). Another study, involving quantitative autoradiographic measurement of binding of ^{3}H-GBR-12935 to the dopamine uptake sites of tissue slices *in vitro*, indicated that aged Fischer 344 rats did not have any change in the density of dopamine uptake sites *per se* in striatum or in several other regions (Inglefield and Richfield, 1992). However, in a study of normal human aging over the range 19 to 100 years, Allard and Marcusson (1989) found an age-related loss of ^{3}H-GBR-12935 uptake sites in putamen. In a comparision of 3-month and 24-month old rats striatal ^{3}H-cocaine binding (to the dopamine transporter) was found to be considerably reduced in the older rats (Govoni *et al.*, 1988).

An age-related decrement in the enhancement of K^+-evoked endogenous dopamine release from rat striatal slices by muscarinic agonists has also been reported (Yamagami *et al.*, 1992) (see also chapter in this volume by El-Fakahany and Joseph). Also there occurs a loss of the capacity of Leu-enkephalin to inhibit K^+-stimulated dopamine release (Lapang *et al.*, 1990), and naloxone or tetrodotoxin treatment appears to restore or reverse the age-related decrement in K^+-evoked dopamine release from rat striatal slices (Dluzen *et al.*, 1988). Gonzales *et al.* (1991) found that the stimulation of ^{3}H-dopamine release from striatal slices of rats by N-methyl-D- aspartate (NMDA) was considerably less in slices from 24-28-month-old Fischer 344 rats than from slices from 12-14-month-old or younger rats.

Haloperidol-induced dopamine turnover in the striatum of C57BL/6J mice was diminished with aging (Severson *et al.*, 1981). Such an effect could be due to an altered presynaptic dopaminergic release process, and/or to a change in postsynaptic striatal mechanisms (e.g., due to decreased dopamine D_2 receptors) and/or to altered strio-nigral mechanisms (Roth and Joseph, 1988; see also below).

Serotonin concentration, synthesis, release and turnover

Serotonin levels generally have been found to be unchanged or moderately increased with senescence in rat brain regions including striatum (Timiras *et al.*, 1982; Van Laijtelaar *et al.*, 1992). There are exceptions to this, however. Thus, Gozlan *et al.* (1990) have reported decreased serotonin content and increased ratio of 5-hydroxyindole acetic acid (5HIAA)/serotonin in hypothalamus, striatum, hippocampus and cerebral cortex of senescent rats. Also Beal *et al.* (1991) reported some non-uniform decreases in serotonin in neocortex of aged rhesus monkeys. No age-related change was found in the number of immunoreactive serotonin neurons in the dorsal raphe of rats (Van Laijtelaar *et al.*, 1992) or C57BL mice (Tatton *et al.*, 1991). We found no impairment of conversion of tryptophan to serotonin by striatal or hypothalamic synaptosomes derived from 24-month-old Fischer 344 rats, compared with that of 12-month-old rats (Makman *et al.*, 1984). In studies of normal (and Alzheimer) human brain neocortical tissue from autopsy brains of age 50-100 years, no significant age-related changes in serotonin uptake or imipramine binding were found (Bowen, 1984). Friedman and Wang (1989) reported age-associated decreases in the rat brain cortex in protein kinase C (PKC) activity, in translocation of PKC in response to K^+-induced depolarization of cortical slices, and in the stimulation of serotonin release from cortical slices by the phorbol ester, phorbol-12-myristate, 13-acetate (an activator of PKC).

Norepinephrine concentration, synthesis, release and turnover

Levels of norepinephrine have generally been found to be not changed or only very moderately changed with aging. Some small decreases in norepinephrine levels and turnover in hypothalamus of senescent male C57BL/J6 mice have been reported (Osterburg *et al.*, 1981). Also there appears to be some (non-uniform) decrease associated with aging in neocortex of rhesus monkeys (Beal *et al.*, 1991) and some region-specific changes in rat brain (Weiland *et al.*, 1989). However, there is no widespread decline in concentration or neuronal activity in female rat brain (Weiland *et al.*, 1989). In marked contrast to those findings, loss of locus coeruleus noradrenergic neurons of C57BL mice from 4 to 104 weeks of age proceeded at a rate even greater than the loss of nigral neurons as discussed above. Thus, by 104 weeks, the number of noradrenergic locus coeruleus neurons had decreased to only 25% of the number at 4 weeks of age (Tatton *et al.*, 1991).

Wise *et al.* (1987) have reported studies of the diurnal pattern of norepinephrine turnover in young and middle-aged ovariectomized estradiol-treated rats. Norepinephrine turnover was measured in median eminence, medial preoptic nucleus and suprachiasmatic nucleus. Norepinephrine turnover was not uniformly decreased in the middle-aged rats. Instead, the primary effect was a diminution of the estradiol-induced diurnal rhythm of norepinephrine turnover (Wise *et al.*, 1987).

NMDA-stimulated ^{3}H-norepinephrine release from hippocampal and cortical slices from Fischer 344 rats decreased with age, although the decrease, particularly in hippocampus, appeared to have occurred already in animals 12-14 months old (Gonzales *et al.*, 1991).

Monoamine receptors

Dopamine receptors

The first studies of age-related changes concerning dopamine receptors were of the dopamine-stimulated adenylate cyclase system (Puri and Volicer, 1977; Schmidt and Thornberry, 1978; Makman *et al.*, 1978), a G_s-coupled system involving dopamine D_1 receptors. Shortly thereafter, aging studies were carried out concerning dopamine D_2 receptors, assessed by radioligand binding studies utilizing ^{3}H-haloperidol or ^{3}H-spiroperidol (Joseph *et al.*, 1978; Makman *et al.*, 1978; Severson and Finch, 1980). Aging studies to the present time have been concerned primarily with these dopaminergic receptor systems, for the most part in striatum, but also in retina, cortex, hypothalamus and certain other brain areas. It should be mentioned that at least two other dopamine receptor subtypes are known and have been cloned, and additional heterogeneity exists as well (Tol *et al.*, 1992). D_2 receptors were first known to be linked to inhibition of adenylate cyclase *via* G_i. However, both D_1 and D_2 receptors may influence the phosphatidyl inositol signal transduction system. Alternative coupling of D_1 receptors to G_s or to G_i (Sidhu *et al.*, 1991) and of D_2 receptors to G_{oa} and to G_{i3a} (Lledo *et al.*, 1992) has been described. Alternative G protein coupling of other receptors, including the β-adrenergic receptor (Okamoto *et al.*, 1991) and δ opioid receptors (McKenzie *et al.*, 1991; Cruciani *et al.*, 1993), has also been observed. These additional considerations of receptor heterogeneity and G protein linkage remain to be taken into consideration in evaluation of the influence of aging on the dopaminergic system.

D_2 receptors

An age-related loss of dopamine D_2 receptors in striatum, measured with antagonist ligand, has been found to occur in striatum of several species including rats, mice, rabbits, rhesus monkeys and humans (Joseph *et al.*, 1978; Makman *et al.*, 1978; Severson and Finch, 1980; Thal *et al.*, 1980; Severson *et al.*, 1982; Hirschhorn *et al.*, 1982; Roth, 1982; Trabucchi *et al.*, 1982; Henry *et al.*, 1986; Joyce *et al.*, 1986; Lai *et al.*, 1987; Morgan and May, 1990). Receptor density (B_{max}) is decreased without change in K_D (usually antagonist affinity only has been evaluated). The overall loss found in these and in a number of additional studies, from young or mid-life to senescence, varies somewhat but in general is in the range of 30%. While this is not an extremely large change, it may be noted that the decrease produced by agonist desensitization, or the increase produced by antagonist administration or denervation, is of about the same magnitude or in some cases even less.

In some studies the decrease in D_2 receptors was already evident by midlife, and appeared to continue thereafter as well. In other studies, loss of D_2 receptors was found to be a process occurring only from mid-life to senescence. Thus, Randall *et al.* (1981) found no loss of striatal D_2 receptors of C57BL/6J mice from 5 to 12 months, followed by a 21% loss from 12 to 24-26 months. While decreases in dopamine metabolism were typically seen only later, with senescence (discussed above) this may be because of compensatory mechanisms; and the loss of dopaminergic neuronal cell bodies may in fact have occurred at the same time as or prior to the loss of dopamine receptors.

Studies were carried out in our laboratory of possible age-related changes in D_2 receptor antagonist (^{3}H-spiroperidol) and agonist (^{3}H- 2-amino-6,7-dihydroxy-1,2,3,4-tetrahydronaphthalene (ADTN)) binding sites in striatum and retina of young (5-6 months of age) and old (5.5 years of age) female New Zealand white rabbits (Makman *et al.*, 1978, 1979, 1980b; Thal *et al.*, 1980). In striatum, antagonist binding was 28% lower and agonist binding 59% lower (a significantly greater change than for antagonist binding) in the old animals, whereas there was no age-related change in the retina.

Govoni *et al.* (1988) compared the density of striatal D_2 receptor sites, with use of ^{3}H-spiroperidol as ligand, in 3-month and 24-month-old rats. Binding was significantly reduced in the older rats; however, a subset of D_2 sites displaced by sulpiride or directly labeled by ^{3}H-sulpiride did not appear to be changed with aging. In contrast, Monelli *et al.* (1990), in autoradiographic studies, have reported age-related decreases in ^{3}H-sulpiride binding in rat striatum with the effect most pronounced in the anterior portion. Whether or not there exist differential effects on aging on subtypes of D_2 receptors or on additional dopamine receptor subtypes (D_3, D_4 etc.) remains to be elucidated.

Fernandez-Ruiz *et al.* (1992) reported sex differences in age-related changes in the dopaminergic system, with comparisons of 2-month and 24-26-month-old Wistar rats (female rats were in estrus): D_2 receptor B_{max} decreased in male striatum by 70%, in female striatum by 32%.

Different strains of mice appear to exhibit significant differences in the decline in D_2 receptor density with age (Morgan and Finch, 1988). In comparative studies of age-related changes in striatal dopamine D_2 receptors in several strains of mice (Leprohon, Greenwood and Cinader, 1987; Greenwood and Cinader, 1991) there appears to be a correlation between the number (B_{max}) of D_2 receptors in young mice of a given strain with the subsequent decline in receptor number with aging. Interestingly, strains with higher numbers of receptors at a young age exhibit the greatest absolute decline at a later age. It may be noted that if the decline were to have been expressed as a percent of the level at a young age, the correlation would probably not be very convincing.

Joyce *et al.* (1986) have examined the age-related loss of Fischer 344 rat striatal dopamine D_2 receptors by quantitative autoradiographic techniques. There was a 36% decrease in receptor binding overall from 3-6 months to 26-28 months of age. The principal age-related decrease occurred in the posterior ventrolateral striatum, the region involved in sensorimotor functions that also show impairment with aging. Also, recent studies indicate that the age-dependent loss of striatal D_2 receptors (with ^{3}H-spiroperidol as ligand) may be more pronounced in the matrix areas than in the striosomes (Amenta *et al.*, 1991).

Severson and Randall (1985) measured both the high and low agonist affinity forms (R_H and R_L) of the D_2 receptor in striatum of the C57BL/6J mouse, with ^{3}H-spiroperidol as radioligand, displaced by dopamine and in the presence or absence of Gpp(NH)p. A 4.8- to 7.8-fold shift in K_i for dopamine was produced by Gpp(NH)p, with no effect of aging on K_i or shift due to the guanine nucleotide analogue. When R_H was expressed as a percent of total receptor (R_H + R_L) there occurred a decrease in R_H from 3 to 12 months of age with no further decrease from 12 to 24 months, while total (R_H + R_L) decreased only from 12 to 24 months (by 24%). However, the absolute amount of R_H did decrease from 12 to 24 months (by 19%), as did the binding of the agonist radioligand ^{3}H-N-propyl-apomorphine (by 14%). These studies did not indicate a selective effect of aging on R_H, but rather suggested that age-related changes in the high and low affinity forms of the receptor may not occur strictly in parallel in mouse striatum. A study of D_2 receptors in human putamen has provided some evidence that R_H is not affected by norman human aging (De Keyser *et al.*, 1990).

Our studies of striatal D_2 agonist (^{3}H-ADTN) and antagonist (^{3}H-spiroperidol) binding as a function of age in the rabbit, described above, revealed a considerably greater age-dependent decrease in agonist R_H than in antagonist R_H + R_L binding. In contrast, in studies carried out with ^{3}H-ADTN in striatum of Fischer 344 rats (Hirschhorn *et al.*, 1982), we found that total high affinity agonist binding (B_{max}) was decreased by 36% in the aged rats (24-26 months old) compared with the young rats (6 months old), i.e., approximately the same decrease with age as has been found for antagonist binding.

D_1 receptors and dopamine-stimulated adenylate cyclase

In addition to the age-related decreases in D_2 receptor density, decreases in striatal dopamine D_1 receptor density also are evident, at least in certain species or animal strains, and appear to occur without changes in antagonist affinity. However, the data for D_1 receptors are more conflicting and there have been fewer satisfactory studies of D_1 receptor binding with respect to aging. An age-associated loss of D_1 receptor binding sites, measured with the antagonist ligand ^{3}H-piflutixol, was reported to occur in striatum of Wistar rats (Henry *et al.*, 1986) but not in Sprague-Dawley rats or in C57BL/6J mice (O'Boyle and Waddington, 1984; Henry *et al.*, 1986). The loss of D_1 receptors in Wistar rats was complete by 12 months of age, in contrast to the loss of D_2 receptors which appeared to be progressive over the entire lifespan (Henry *et al.*, 1986). Battaglia and Creese found that the B_{max} for ^{3}H-piflutixol binding in striatum of Fischer 344 rats at 28 months of age was 22% less than at 4 months of age. Hyttel (1987) studied D_1 receptors using the highly selective antagonist ligand ^{3}H-SCH 23390 (a preferable ligand because of lower non-specific binding and greater stability). In this study of striatal binding in Wistar rats from 1 to 12 months of age (but unfortunately not including older rats in the study), a gradual decrease in B_{max} was found with the value at 12 months 35% less than that at 1 month. During this period D_2 receptor binding increased slightly from 1 to 3 months and then declined to a value at 12 months that was 20% lower than the 1-month value. Georgi *et al.* (1987), in a study of D_1 receptors in striatum of Sprague-Dawley rats, also utilized ^{3}H- SCH 23390 and reported findings quite different from those cited above for Sprague-Dawley rats using ^{3}H-piflutixol as ligand. Georgi *et al.* found no significant decrease in striatal D_1 binding from 3 to 14 months of age, although there was a downward trend. However, D_1 receptor density at 20 months was decreased significantly, by 37% compared to the 3-month value and by 29% compared to the 14-month value; also the value at 26 months was decreased by 44% compared to the 3-month value and by 33% compared to the 20-month value. Also in a recent study using ^{3}H-SCH 23390 as ligand, there appeared to be essentially equivalent losses with age of D_1 and D_2 receptors in human brain (Rinne *et al.*, 1990).

In recent autoradiographic studies with ^{3}H-SCH 23390 as ligand, D_1 receptor density was found to be reduced particularly in the anterior portion of the striatum of male Sprague-Dawley rats at 24 months of age (Monelli *et al.*, 1990).

Also, Amenta *et al.* (1991) reported that age-dependent loss of rat striatal D_1 receptors involved both the matrix and the striosomes but was more pronounced in the matrix, as was the case also for loss of D_2 receptors.

Early studies by Puri and Volicer (1977) and Schmidt and Thornberry (1978) indicated that D_1 receptor-mediated stimulation of adenylate cyclase activity of rat striatum was decreased in senescent animals. Puri and Volicer (1977) studied adenylate cyclase activity of the striatum of Sprague-Dawley rats at ages 4, 12, 24 and 30 months of age. The maximal stimulation of activity by dopamine at 4 months was about 55%. No age-related change in basal or NaF-stimulated activity was found. Dopamine-stimulated adenylate cyclase activity decreased throughout the lifespan of the animals, with essentially no stimulation by dopamine evident at 30 months of age. These results correlate with the D_1 antagonist radioligand binding studies of Georgi *et al.* (1987), described above. However, other studies of rat striatal activity, including our own studies of Fischer 344 rats described below, have yielded different results. A number of factors may contribute to the differences in findings of various investigators for age-related changes in D_1 receptor-mediated stimulation of adenylate cyclase, as discussed later. Possibly, differences are at least in part due to the strain of rat used. Thus, Schmidt and Thornberry (1978) studied striatal adenylate cyclase activity of Wistar rats at ages 3, 12 and 24 months. At maximally effective concentrations, dopamine caused about a doubling of activity at 3 months of age. There occurred about a 20% decline in the stimulation of activity by dopamine from 2 to 12 months, with no further decline noted at 24 months.

Our laboratory carried out studies of dopamine-stimulated adenylate cyclase activity of striatum of male Fischer 344 rats at 4.5, 14 and 29 months of age, as well as female rats at 14 and 29 months of age (Hirschhorn *et al.*, 1982; Makman *et al.*, 1984). Dopamine at maximally effective concentrations caused at least a doubling of activity at all ages and there was no age-related change in stimulation by dopamine.

Our laboratory has also investigated possible age-related changes in amine receptor–adenylate cyclase activity in brain regions and retina of young (5-6 months of age) and old (5.5 years of age) female New Zealand white rabbits (Makman *et al.*, 1978, 1979, 1980a, 1980b). The brain regions studied, striatum, hypothalamus, anterior limbic cortex and frontal cortex, are regions which have been thought to be particularly involved in human brain aging. The rabbit brain provides a source of adenylate cyclases which we have found to be generally more stable and sensitive to transmitters than is the case for several other experimental animals (e.g., rat and mouse) more commonly used in aging studies. For example, dopamine increased the activity of striatal membranes of young rabbits to a value about three times the basal level. No age-related difference between the young and old animals was found for basal activity or for the marked stimulation of activity by Gpp(NH)p in any of the four brain regions studied or in retina. The increments in adenylate cyclase activities due to the presence of dopamine over a range of concentrations was significantly decreased in the old animals in each of the four brain regions studied. In each of the brain regions the age-related decrease clearly involved the maximal effectiveness of dopamine, which was reduced by about 40%. However, an additional component involving reduced sensitivity to dopamine was suggested by the even greater differences found at lower dopamine concentrations. The effects of aging in the cortex and hypothalamus were not entirely selective for dopamine, since histamine-stimulated adenylate cyclase, a highly active system in frontal cortex, anterior limbic cortex and hypothalamus of the young rabbits, was also decreased in the older animals. The decrease in histamine-stimulated activity was about the same extent as that observed for dopamine. Not all dopamine-stimulated systems were affected by aging, however, since the dopamine-stimulated adenylate cyclase of retina showed no difference at all between the young and old animals.

Amenta *et al.* (1990) have reported an age-related decrease in dopamine-stimulated adenylate cyclase activity in rat frontal cortex. The decrease in this instance appeared to have occurred already by midlife.

It appears that age-related decreases in dopamine-stimulated adenylate cyclase in some instances may already be evident by midlife, and in other instances may occur (or continue to occur) later in the lifespan, while in still other instances no change may be evident. At least in some instances changes clearly occur and are of a magnitude at least comparable to the magnitude of changes in dopamine receptor binding (D_1 and D_2). In view of the differences found in the various studies, it seems likely that not only are strain or species differences involved, but also the state of the animal and presence or absence of various compensatory factors may be particularly important. For example, possibly less dopamine release or other presynaptic changes in the intact animal may lead to compensatory increases in dopamine-stimulated cyclase ("supersensitivity") that counterbalance an age-related decrease (see below).

Murray and Waddington (1991) studied age-related changes in the regulation of behavior involving interactions between a dopamine D_1 (SCH 23390) and a D_2 receptor agonist (LY 163502) administered *in vivo* to Sprague-Dawley rats. These investigators also measured D_2 and D_1 receptor binding in striatum. As in their earlier studies (O'Boyle and

Waddington, 1984), only D_2 receptor density decreased with age and even the D_2 receptor effect was less than has generally been observed. However, the behavioral results indicated that the net effect of aging was to reduce tonic activity through D_1 receptors to a greater extent than through D_2 receptors. Possible explanations considered by the investigators were that the responsible mechanism might be either a presynaptic mechanism or a postsynaptic mechanism beyond the D_1 receptor itself. Since D_1 receptor–agonist interactions were not evaluated, it may be that the postsynaptic site is at the level of receptor-G protein coupling or other site close to if not actually the D_1 receptor itself.

Porceddu *et al.* (1990) have carried out an interesting study of dopamine D_1 antagonist binding and dopamine-stimulated adenylate cyclase activity in retinas of rats at 3, 14 and 26 months of age. For animals in the normal lighted environment, B_{max} values for ^{3}H-SCH-23390 binding were increased by 34% at 14 months and by 73% at 26 months when compared to the 3-month-old rats. Also, aging failed to alter sensitivity or maximal stimulatory effect of dopamine on adenylate cyclase. However, when animals were dark-adapted, the old animals exhibited no change in dopamine-stimulated adenylate cyclase and no further change in D_1 antagonist binding. In contrast, the young animals upon dark adaptation exhibited the expected increase in retinal ^{3}H-SCH-23390 binding and in dopamine-stimulated adenylate cyclase activity. Thus, for the older animals, retinal binding sites appear to be fixed in an enhanced state, the same as that of the young animals after dark adaptation, whether or not the animals are in the dark. However, for the older animals, the response of adenylate cyclase to dopamine appears to remain or be fixed in the "light-desensitized" state and unable to resensitize when the animals are put in the dark. The findings suggest that receptor coupling as well as receptor turnover are involved in the normal light-adaptation process. The basis for the age-related changes remains to be elucidated. Clearly, the responsiveness of the system is lost with aging.

Dopamine receptor supersensitivity and desensitization

Randall *et al.* (1981) examined the influence of aging on the ability of the dopamine antagonist haloperidol to induce receptor "up-regulation" in C57BL/6J mice. Chronic treatment of 5-month-old mice with haloperidol followed by withdrawal of the drug led to an expected 27% increase in B_{max} for striatal D_2 (^{3}H-spiroperidol) binding. There was no change at 12 months, but at 24-26 months there was no longer a significant up-regulation due to haloperidol treatment. In contrast, chronic treatment with the dopamine agonist bromocriptine led to decreased binding ("down-regulation") in all age groups.

It appears that binding of the high affinity agonist (^{3}H-ADTN) to D_2 receptors can be resolved further into two saturable components, a component that is lost upon addition of Gpp(NH)p (Gpp(NH)p-sensitive component) and another component still evident in the presence of Gpp(NH)p (Gpp(NH)p-insensitive component) (Hirschhorn *et al.*, 1980; Makman *et al.*, 1982, 1984). Following lesion of the nigrostriatal dopaminergic pathway of young rats with 6-hydroxydopamine, there is a more pronounced increase in B_{max} for ^{3}H-ADTN binding sites than is generally found for ^{3}H-spiroperidol binding; in addition, there is a considerably greater increase in the Gpp(NH)p-sensitive than in the Gpp(NH)p-insensitive component of ^{3}H-ADTN binding (Hirschhorn *et al.*, 1982; Makman *et al.*, 1984). Thus, dopaminergic denervation of young Sprague-Dawley and Fischer 344 rats leads to a particularly large increase in agonist binding sites highly coupled to (and hence sensitive to) guanine nucleotide regulation. Following dopaminergic denervation of the old Fischer 344 rats (24 months of age), Gpp(NH)p-insensitive ^{3}H-ADTN binding exhibited about the same % increase (85%) as occurred in the young rats (6 months of age) (74%) due to denervation. However, the old rats exhibited a marked impairment in response to denervation with respect to guanine nucleotide-sensitive binding. No change at all was found in the old rats, while there was a 134% increase in young rats due to denervation (Hirschhorn *et al.*, 1982).

We propose that in the intact young rat there probably exists a tonic "down-regulation" of guanine nucleotide-sensitive ^{3}H-ADTN binding sites that is reversed by denervation. Therefore, it may be the reversal of this down-regulation that is actually defective in the aged rats. Whether or not new synthesis of receptors is needed for this reversal is not known (see also below). It may also be noted that the "new" intrinsic striatal D_2 receptors present in young animals following denervation bind both ^{3}H-spiroperidol and ^{3}H-ADTN. The affinity of ADTN for these new sites (agonist affinity) is appreciably greater than the overall affinity of ADTN for D_2 sites in the intact striatum (Makman *et al.*, 1984).

Denervation of the rat nigrostriatal dopaminergic pathway also leads to an enhanced dopamine-stimulated adenylate cyclase (Mishra *et al.*, 1974), amounting to about a doubling of the usual stimulation by dopamine in intact striatum. In our studies of the influence of aging on striatal adenylate cyclase in the Fischer 344 rat, not only was there no age-related decrease in stimulation by dopamine of activity in intact striatum, as indicated above, but also dopamine-stimulated activity was enhanced equally by denervation in the young and the old rats (Hirschhorn *et al.*, 1982).

Mechanisms for age-related changes in dopamine receptors

The loss of D_2 receptors in aged animals does not appear to be due to or accompanied by internalization of receptors (Roth and Josephs, 1988). The loss does not appear to occur in aged rats that have been placed on a restricted diet (Levin *et al.*, 1981), a finding that argues against the loss of D_2 receptors being due to intrinsic strictly programmed factor(s). The rate of loss of striatal D_2 receptors following irreversible inactivation *in vivo* and also the rate of recovery (resynthesis) following inactivation has been studied in young and aged rats (Henry *et al.*, 1984). There was no difference in the rate of loss of D_2 receptors in the senescent rats; however, the rate of recovery was decreased by 25-35% in the senescent rats. In analogous studies of rat striatal D_1 receptors, following *in vivo* receptor inactivation, there was also an age-related decrease in the recovery rate of D_1 receptors (Battaglia *et al.*, 1988). Thus, decreased rate of receptor synthesis may be one factor contributing to decreases in D_1 and D_2 receptor density found with aging, with the decreases in D_1 receptor density possibly also accounting for changes in dopamine-stimulated adenylate cyclase. It should be pointed out that a decreased rate of synthesis in turn might be due to one of several factors, including a selective change in receptor synthesis within the neuron, or a decrease in the number of neurons capable of synthesizing the receptors.

While parallel changes in the dopamine receptor subtypes and dopamine-stimulated adenylate cyclase have not been observed in some studies, the reason for this is not clear. Apart from technical factors that may lead to misleading results, it may be that a common underlying cause is obscured by additional interactions that are selective for a receptor subtype and/or the adenylate cyclase system.

Serotonin receptors

Bowen (1984), in studies of normal human neocortical tissue, found an age-related decrease in $5HT_2$ receptor density from about 50 years of age and especially marked by 80 years. Gozlan *et al.* (1990) have reported age-related decreases in male rat brain regions (dentate, cortex, substantia nigra, striatum) of serotonin $5HT_{1B}$ receptors, a smaller loss of $5HT_2$ receptors and no loss of $5HT_{1A}$ receptors; the loss of $5HT_{1B}$ was somewhat less than that of striatal dopamine D_2 receptors. In our studies of ^3H-spiroperidol binding to $5HT_2$ receptor sites in cortex of young (5-6 months of age) and old (5.5 years of age) female New Zealand white rabbits, binding was decreased significantly in both frontal cortex (–30%) and in anterior limbic cortex (–21%) (Makman *et al.*, 1978, 1979, 1980b; Thal *et al.*, 1980).

α-adrenergic and β-adrenergic receptors

Greenberg and Weiss (1979) have reported an age-related decrease in β-adrenergic receptor density (measured with ^{3}H-dihydroalprenolol) in rat brain. An additional and striking finding was that aged rats had a considerably diminished ability to increase β-adrenergic receptor density in cerebral cortex, cerebellum and pineal gland following repeated administration of reserpine. In contrast, there was no impairment of the ability of aged rats to decrease β-adrenergic receptor density in response to desmethylimipramine.

No age-related changes were found for β-adrenergic (^{3}H-dihydroalprenolol) receptor binding in neocortex or caudate of normal (or Alzheimer) human brain tissue (autopsy brains of age 50-100 years) (Bowen, 1984). In a recent study (Kalaria *et al.*, 1992) a significant age-related decrease was found for α_2-adrenergic (^{3}H-p-aminoclonidine) receptor binding in normal human prefrontal cortex, with an additional loss associated with Alzheimer's disease. A decrease in α_1 receptor density, assessed with ^{3}H-prazosin as ligand, has been reported to occur in medial preoptic nucleus and median eminence of aged female rats in a state of persistent pseudopregnancy, but not in estrus/diestrus or constant estrus animals (Weiland *et al.*, 1989).

Presynaptic–postsynaptic dopaminergic interrelationships

Postsynaptic age-related changes may no doubt be influenced by presynaptic changes. It seems likely that presynaptic dopaminergic neuronal loss, to the extent that it is not compensated for, would tend to mask postsynaptic losses of dopamine receptors by up-regulation of the remaining receptors. The cholinergic, GABAergic and opioid systems are closely interrelated with the dopamine system in the striatum. Cell types in striatum containing D_1 and/or D_2 receptors include most likely cholinergic and also GABAergic interneurons. GABAergic neurons project from striatum to globus pallidus and to substantia nigra, and at least the nigral projection contains D_1 receptors. Also, D_2 receptors may be on nerve terminals in striatum of glutaminergic neurons projecting from cortex to striatum. There is no convincing evidence overall for loss of these neurons directly accounting for the age-related decreases in striatal dopaminergic receptor systems, and the same probably holds true for dopaminergic systems in other brain regions. In some species presynaptic cholinergic and GABAergic markers may be altered, however, and a few studies indicate postsynaptic changes. The reader is referred to Chapter 2 by Carpenter *et al.* and Chapter 3 by El-Fakahany and Joseph for further consideration of the cholinergic system, and to Chapter 8 by Bodnar and Pasternak and Chapter 10 by Stefano for further consideration of the opioid system. It may be noted that Bowen (1984) in studies of normal human autopsy brains of age 50-100 years found in neocortex and caudate nucleus age-related decrease in choline acetyltransferase, a cholinergic presynaptic marker, from about 50 years of age and especially marked by 80 years. In contrast, there was no change in cholinergic muscarinic (quinuclidinyl benzilate) binding or in ^{3}H-naloxone binding to opioid receptors. In our studies of age-related changes in rabbit brain described above, the changes in dopaminergic systems were not accompanied by any changes in choline acetyltransferase activity or in muscarinic cholinergic receptor binding (Makman *et al.*, 1978, 1980a). An age-related decrease in rat striatal choline acetyltransferase, particularly from 5 to 13 months of age, has been reported by Sims *et al.* (1982). Also, age-related decrease in acetylcholine synthesis in mouse striatum *in vivo* has been reported by Gibson and Peterson (1982).

Bowen (1984), in studies of normal human autopsy brains found age-related decrease in GABA uptake in neocortex and glutamate decarboxylase in the entire temporal lobe, as well as increased concentration of glutamate in neocortex and increased muscimol binding in temporal lobe. Synthesis of GABA from glucose is decreased in brain of senescent C57BL mice (Gibson and Peterson, 1982). The influence of aging on release of amino acids from rat brain synaptosomes prelabeled with ^{14}C-aspartate, ^{14}C-glutamate and ^{14}C-GABA has been studied using synaptosomes from 4-6-month-old and from 24-26-month-old rats (Aprikyan and Gekchyan, 1988). Decreased K^{+}-stimulated release of all three amino acids was found using synaptosomes from the older animals, with both Ca^{2+}-dependent and Ca^{2+}-independent release affected by aging.

Adenylate cyclase, other signal transduction systems and G proteins

Age-related decreases in dopamine-stimulated adenylate cyclase activity, as reviewed above, were not accompanied by changes in basal activity or in activity measured in the presence of forskolin or guanine nucleotide analogues. The evidence thus far is against any global changes in catalytic activity of adenylate cyclase or in G proteins linked to adenylate cyclase. Possible changes in the G protein coupling of specific receptors to adenylate cyclase has essentially not been evaluated as a causative factor for changes in transmitter-modulated adenylate cyclase. Also, there is little information concerning the status of specific G proteins in the aged animal.

There is relatively little information available concerning the status of signal transduction systems, other than adenylate cyclase, in the aged animal. Undie and Friedman (1992) have recently reported a study of age-related changes in phosphoinositide (PI) metabolism of brain tissue slices from 6-month-old and 24-month-old Fischer 344 rats. In addition to altered basal turnover of the inositol cycle, it was found for the old rats that there was a decreased ability of the dopamine D_1 agonist, SKF 38393, to stimulate the formation of inositol phosphates in striatal, hippocampal and frontal cerebral cortical slices. Thus, functional coupling of dopamine D_1 receptors not only to adenylate cyclase, but also to PI metabolism, appears to be decreased with aging in rat brain. An age-related decrease in stimulation of inositol phosphate formation in cortical slices by the muscarinic cholinergic agonist carbachol has also been reported (Kurian *et al.*, 1992). There appears to be at least some degree of specificity for age-related changes with respect to transmitter and region. A relatively small but significant age-related decrease in receptor for inositol 1,4,5-trisphosphate has also been reported to occur in rat cerebellum (Li *et al.*, 1992).

Battaini *et al.* (1990) have reported a decrease in ^{3}H-phorbol-12,13-dibutyrate binding, presumably to protein kinase C, in rat brain cortex with age. Also, changes in protein kinase C have been reported to occur in rat cortex with aging (Friedman and Wang, 1987; see also discussion of serotonin release above).

Calcium ion plays a central role in signal transduction generally, as well as in neurotransmission at many levels. The roles of Ca^{2+} in signal transduction include modulation of calmodulin-dependent adenylate cyclase, phosphodiesterases and protein kinases, influences on protein kinase C and mobilization of intracellular calcium stores. The reader is referred to Chapter 5 by Satrústegui *et al.* for discussion of Ca^{2+} and aging. It may be noted here that some studies have indicated impaired calcium availability and decreased calcium uptake with aging, including impaired basal and K^+-induced Ca^{2+} uptake by forebrain synaptosomes from Fischer 344 rats (Gibson and Peterson, 1987; Gibson *et al.*, 1987). Some studies of age-related changes in monoamine release, referred to above, suggest possible loss of calcium-dependent processes. In addition, a number of studies, including those of Satrústegui and collaborators, indicate increased free Ca^{2+} in aged brain. Massie *et al.* (1989) found that total calcium content of brain increased with aging in C57BL/6J mice. Michaelis *et al.* (1992), in studies of whole rat brain synaptosomes, monitoring intrasynaptosomal Ca^{2+} with fura-2, reported that resting [Ca^{2+}] (about 200 nM) was the same in synaptosomes from adult (5-8 months) and aged (23-25 months) rats. However, the increase in [Ca^{2+}] upon depolarization with KCl, veratridine or ibotenic acid was greater in synaptosomes from aged animals. Also, total calcium content of synaptosomes and whole brain was greater for the aged rats. Hence there may be more calcium to be mobilized upon depolarization, and certain calcium responses may be facilitated in neurons of aged animals (e.g., see Landfield and Pitler, 1984). Overall, regulation by calcium appears to be impaired with aging.

Age-related changes in monoamine systems in peripheral tissues: age-related changes in the myocardium and comparison with the CNS

To attempt a detailed review of age-related changes in all peripheral monoaminergic systems is beyond the scope of this chapter. As in the CNS, age-related changes in the peripheral nervous system and their target tissues appear to be non-uniform and rather selective. We will consider here those changes in the myocardium that relate to β-adrenergic responsiveness. In association with normal aging in man as well as in experimental animals, a number of changes in myocardial function have been documented, including decreased β-adrenergic myocardial responsiveness (Filburn and Lakatta, 1987; Lakatta, 1990). In isolated rat cardiac muscle or perfused heart muscle preparations, there is an age-related decrement in the inotropic effect of β-adrenergic agonists, without a shortening of the contraction duration. Mechanisms proposed to account for the age-related changes have included possible decreases in high affinity β-adrenergic binding sites for agonist, diminished β-adrenergic-stimulated adenylate cyclase, diminished G protein coupling, as well as age-related changes distal to the adenylate cyclase system (Lakatta, 1990).

Studies of adenylate cyclase activity of rat myocardium by Scarpace and coworkers (O'Connor *et al.*, 1981; Scarpace, 1990) have indicated that age-associated decreases in stimulation of activity by β-adrenergic agonist and by forskolin occur. In an early study (Narayanan and Derby, 1982), a diminished receptor coupling *via* G protein was proposed, based on elimination of the age-related difference by addition of guanine nucleotides. However, another study of the effects of GTP analogues on myocardial activity suggests that the age-related changes are due to a decrease in catalytic activity independent of the presence or absence of activated G protein (Scarpace, 1990).

Chevalier *et al.* (1991) have compared the receptor densities for left ventricular β-adrenergic receptors (^{125}I-iodocyanopindolol as ligand) and muscarinic receptor (^{3}H-quinuclidinyl benzilate as ligand) of male Wistar rats at 4 months and 24 months of age. B_{max} values for β-adrenergic and for muscarinic receptors were decreased by 26% and 48% respectively in the old rats. Interestingly, continuous infusion of propranolol or atropine up-regulated the β-adrenergic and muscarinic receptor densities in the aged but not in the young adult rats, thereby apparently reversing the effects of aging. The authors conclude that the changes in receptors with aging are reversible and can return to adult levels by chronic administration of appropriate antagonist. These results imply that in the aged animals the decrease in myocardial receptors is due to enhanced tonic level of down-regulation, either *via* enhanced sympathetic and parasympathetic activity or alternatively *via* intrinsically altered (enhanced) myocardial responses to sympathetic and parasympathetic activity, which antagonist administration can then override.

We have recently carried out studies of age-related changes in the adenylate cyclase system of myocardial membranes and in cyclic AMP concentrations of isolated cardiomyocytes obtained from Fischer 344 rats. We have also investigated the influence of age of the rat on calcium ion concentration ([Ca^{2+}]) in the isolated cardiomyocytes.

Table 1. Influence of Aging on Adenylate Cyclase of Left Ventricular Tissue

Age (months)	(n)	Activity (pmoles cyclic AMP formed/mg protein)			
		basal	isoproterenol (10 μM)	secretin (1 μM)	forskolin (10 μM)
2 - 5	(8)	33 ± 3	180 ± 8	335 ± 18	336 ± 12
6 - 11	(4)	31 ± 2	158 ± 8	219 ± 12	316 ± 14
16 - 20	(6)	28 ± 3	180 ± 9	183 ± 6	266 ± 11
23 - 26	(5)	21 ± 2	106 ± 7	76 ± 4	169 ± 7

Age-associated decreases, based on absolute stimulation, were found for secretin-stimulated as well as for β-adrenergic agonist (isoproterenol)- and forskolin-stimulated adenylate cyclase activity of ventricular and papillary muscle tissues (Tables 1 and 2). Basal activity also decreased with age in both ventricular and papillary muscle preparations. The % stimulation by isoproterenol above basal activity was not changed with age in ventricular muscle but did decrease significantly in papillary muscle. Percent stimulation by secretin as well as the absolute amount of stimulation was decreased with age in both muscle preparations. Inhibition of the forskolin-activated adenylate cyclase of papillary muscle by the muscarinic agonist carbachol was not significantly changed (slightly increased) with age (Table 2).

Table 2. Influence of Aging on Adenylate Cyclase of Rat Papillary Muscle Tissue

Age (months)	(n)	Activity (pmoles cyclic AMP formed/mg protein				
		basal	isoproterenol (10 μM)	secretin (1 μM)	forskolin (10 μM)	forskolin (10 μM) + carbachol (10 μM)
2 - 5	(9)	58 ± 2	450 ± 18	554 ± 21	855 ± 30	666 ± 32
6 - 11	(4)	23 ± 2	192 ± 11	199 ± 9	575 ± 28	491 ± 27
16 - 20	(6)	36 ± 2	179 ± 7	182 ± 8	421 ± 17	330 ± 22
23 - 26	(7)	30 ± 2	148 ± 5	54 ± 3	454 ± 20	308 ± 18

The component of adenylate cyclase activated by secretin was found also to be activated by the structurally related proteins glucagon and vasoactive intestinal peptide (VIP). These peptides all appear to interact at the same receptor site, a site distinct from that influenced by the β-adrenergic agonists. Age-related decreases in VIP-stimulated adenylate cyclase and, to a lesser extent, in glucagon-stimulated cyclase of ventricular muscle tissue were also found to occur (data not shown).

Isolated ventricular heart muscle cells and whole ventricular tissue contain approximately the same levels of adenylate cyclase activity (data not shown). Cyclic AMP concentrations in intact myocytes, and stimulation of cyclic AMP by isoproterenol and forskolin, were found to be markedly decreased in myocytes from the aged animals (Table 3). Isolated ventricular fibroblasts contain only about 25-30% of the activity present in the isolated cardiomyocytes (measured in the presence of isoproterenol or forskolin). Interestingly, isolated ventricular fibroblasts contain an adenylate cyclase system that is activated by glucagon as well as by isoproterenol. In contrast to the results for cardiomyocytes, the adenylate cyclase of the isolated fibroblasts appears to be the same in cells from 4-5-month and from 24-25-month-old animals (data not shown).

Table 3. Influence of Donor Age on Cyclic AMP Levels in Intact Rat Cardiomyocytes.

Additions to cell incubation for 5 min*	Cyclic AMP level (pmoles/mg protein) Young: 3 - 4 months	Old: 23 - 24 months	Ratio: young/old
Basal (none)	25.0 ± 0.7	8.0 ± 0.4	0.32
Norepinephrine, 10 μM	78.4 ± 2.4	18.3 ± 0.9	0.23
Isoproterenol, 10 μM	68.0 ± 3.3	23.6 ± 1.1	0.35
Forskolin, 10 μM	189.5 ± 9.3	35.6 ± 1.2	0.19

* Incubations in presence of isobutyl-methylxanthine

For measurement of intracellular [Ca^{2+}], purified myocytes were first loaded with the acetylmethoxy ester of fura-2 (fura-2-AM), then washed, and [Ca^{2+}] of the cell suspensions determined by standard fluorometric procedures. Generally, after establishing basal levels of [Ca^{2+}], the influence of elevated potassium ion or various other agents added to the same cell suspension could then be assessed. Important variables include the concentration of calcium ion in which the myocytes are finally isolated (prior to loading with fura-2-AM) and the concentration of extracellular calcium ion present during the actual measurements of intracellular [Ca^{2+}]. Myocytes purified from hearts of 4-5-month-old Fischer 344 rats, when isolated in 0.3 mM Ca^{2+}, had a higher basal and KCl-stimulated intracellular [Ca^{2+}] than did myocytes made "tolerant" to calcium by final step up from 0.3 mM to 1.0 mM Ca^{2+} and equilibration in the 1.0 mM Ca^{2+}. Intracellular [Ca^{2+}] was investigated in myocytes from rats 24-25 months of age, as well as in cells from the younger animals (Table 4). Interestingly, myocytes from the older rats not only had highly stable basal [Ca^{2+}], but basal levels were even slightly lower than in the younger animals (difference, however, not statistically significant). Furthermore, in the presence of 50 mM KCl, [Ca^{2+}] was significantly lower in the old than in the young myocyte preparation. These studies indicate that the myocytes from the older animals are equivalent to those from the younger animals in terms of intactness, stability and presence of a physiologically normal intracellular calcium ion concentration. In view of these results concerning intracellular [Ca^{2+}], the finding of major alterations in the capacity of the older myocytes to form cyclic AMP takes on added significance.

Table 4. Intracellular Calcium Ion Concentration in Rat Ventricular Myocytes

Preparation	Intracellular [Ca^{2+}], nM	
	Basal	+50 mM KCl
	(extracellular [Ca^{2+}] = 2.4mM)	
4-5 months old; cells isolated in 0.3 mM Ca^{2+}	190 ± 23	385 ± 44
4-5 months old; cells isolated in 1.0 mM Ca^{2+}	131 ± 12	231 ± 20
24-25 months old; cells isolated in 1.0 mM Ca^{2+}	98 ± 9	190 ± 13
	(extracellular [Ca^{2+}] = 1.0 mM)	
4-5 months old; cells isolated in 1.0 mM Ca^{2+}	56 ± 5	188 ± 11
24-25 months old; cells isolated in 1.0 mM Ca^{2+}	9 ± 3	142 ± 6

Values are means ± S.E.M.s (n = 4 - 7)

The basic alterations in myocardial ß-adrenergic receptors and adenylate cyclase bear some resemblance to the alterations in β-adrenergic and also dopaminergic alterations in the central nervous system, even though there are also differences in the specific age-related changes. One common theme is the existence of age-related changes in the status of receptors in terms of up-regulation and/or down-regulation, possibly a reflection of the ability of receptors to be modulated by external factors (Chevalier *et al.*, 1991; Greenberg and Weiss, 1979; Randall *et al.*, 1981; Makman *et al.*, 1984; Porceddu *et al.*, 1990). It is of interest that the end result in terms of monoaminergic responsiveness of these different systems in the aged animal may be the same, even though the detailed molecular changes involved in achieving that result may be different. The age-related modifications in adenylate cyclase and G proteins clearly do not follow any single pattern in the different systems investigated. Yet here again, the end result, decreased overall functional coupling of receptor to second messenger system, may be the same in certain brain regions and the myocardium.

Conclusions and directions for future study

The central dopaminergic, noradrenergic and serotonergic systems appear to be differentially affected by the aging process, with further differences most likely existing within discrete anatomical and functional units. If indeed there are major age-associated losses of discrete monoaminergic cell populations, as indicated by studies cited in this chapter, then there must also be major compensatory presynaptic mechanisms operating as well. These compensatory mechanisms must be very efficient for the noradrenergic system, since there appears to be relatively little functional deficit at the noradrenergic nerve terminal. More complex compensatory changes may occur at the dopaminergic nerve terminal, and the serotonergic system appears to be relatively spared such age-related changes. Postsynaptic changes, including alterations in receptor-signal transduction systems, are probably in part primary and in part secondary in response to presynaptic alterations. Sequences of events and primary causes at this point are essentially unknown. Underlying molecular bases for age-related changes are also for the most part entirely unknown. However, the observed changes in central monoaminergic function do account for the extent and nature of functional deficits in brain function associated with normal human aging. It should be possible in future studies to obtain a better understanding of the molecular mechanisms underlying these changes, as well as the causal relationships among the changes. Similar considerations apply to the myocardium. Such understanding should provide the basis for more rational and effective pharmacotherapy and more generally the clinical management of the elderly patient.

Acknowledgements

This work was supported in part by a National Institutes of Health Grant AG05554.

References

Allard, P. and Marcusson, J. O. (1989). Age-correlated loss of dopamine uptake sites labeled with [^{3}H]GBR-12935 in human putamen. *Neurobiol. Aging* **10**: 661-664.

Amenta, F., Cacallotti, C., Collier, W. L., de Michele, M. and Ricci, A. (1990). Age-related changes of dopamine-sensitive cyclic AMP generation in the rat frontal cortex. *Mech. Ageing Dev.* **54**: 63-73.

Amenta, F., Zaccheo, D. and Collier, W. L. (1991). Neurotransmitters, neuroreceptors and aging. *Mech. Ageing Dev.* **61**: 249-273.

Aprikyan, G. V. and Gekchyan, K. G. (1988). Release of neurotransmitter amino acids from rat brain synaptosomes and its regulation in aging. *Gerontolgy* **34**: 35-40.

Ayd, F. J. (1961). A survey of drug-induced extra-pyramidal reactions. *J. Amer. Med. Ass.* **175**: 1054-1060.

Battaglia, G., Norman, A. B. and Creese, I. (1988). Age-related differential recovery rates of striatal D-1 dopamine receptors following irreversible inactivation. *Eur. J. Pharmacol.* **145**: 281-290.

Battaini, F., Del Vesco, R., Govoni, S. and Trabucchi, M. (1990). Regulation of phorbol ester binding and protein kinase C activity in aged brain. *Neurobiol. Aging* **11**: 563-566.

Beal, M. F., Walker, L. C., Storey, E., Segar, L., Price, D. L. and Cork, L. C. (1991). Neurotransmitters in neocortex of aged rhesus monkeys. *Neurobiol. Aging* **12**: 407-412.

Bowen, D. M. (1984). Cellular ageing: selective vulnerability of cholinergic neurons in human brain. *Monogr. Dev. Biol.* **17**: 42-59. Chapter in: *Cellular Ageing*, ed. Sauer, H. W., Karger, Basel, 1984.

Carlsson, A. (1987) Brain neurotransmitters in aging and dementia: similar changes across diagnostic dementia groups. *Gerontology* 33: 159-167.

Chevalier, B., Mansier, P., Teiger, E., Callens-El Amrani, F. and Swynghedauw, B. (1991). Alterations in β-adrenergic and muscarinic receptors in aged rat heart: effects of chronic administration of propranolol and atropine. *Mech. Ageing Dev.* **60**: 215-224.

Cruciani, R. A., Dvorkin, B., Morris, S. A., Crain, S. M. and Makman, M. H. (1993). Direct coupling of opioid receptors to both G_s and G_i proteins in F-11 neuroblastoma × sensory neuron hybrid cells. *Proc. Nat. Acad. Sci. U.S.A.* **90**: 3019-3023.

De Keyser, J., Ebinger, G. and Vauquelin, G. (1990) Age-related changes in the human nigrostriatal dopaminergic system. *Ann. Neurol.* **27**: 157-161.

Dluzen, D. E., Laping, N. J. and Ramirez, V. D. (1988) The importance of striatal interneurons in age related effects upon potassium- and amphetamine-stimulated dopamine release. *Brain Res.* **445**: 354-357.

Fernandez-Ruiz, J., De Miguel, R., Hernandez, M. L., Cebeira, M. and Ramos, J. A. (1992). Comparisons between brain dopaminergic neurons of juvenile and aged rats: sex-related differences. *Mech. Ageing Dev.* **63**: 45-55.

Filburn, C. R. and Lakatta, E. G. (1987). Aged related alterations in the β-adrenergic modulation of cardiac cell function. Chapter in: *Aging and Cell Function*, ed. Johnson, J. E., New York, Plenum Press, pp. 211-238.

Finch, C. E. (1973). Catecholamine metabolism in the brains of aging male mice. *Brain Res.* **52**: 261-276.

Friedman, E. and Wang, H. Y. (1989). Effect of age on brain cortical protein kinase C and its mediation of 5-hydroxytryptamine release. *J. Neurochem.* **52**: 187-192.

Friedmann, M. N. and Gerhardt, G. A. (1992) Regional effects of aging on dopaminergic function in the Fischer-344 rat. *Neurobiol. Aging* **13**: 325-332.

Garber, S. L. and Makman, M. H. (1987). Regulation of tryptophan hydroxylase activity by a cyclic AMP-dependent mechanism in rat striatum. *Molec. Brain Res.* 3: 1-10.

Gibson, G. E. and Peterson, C. (1982). Biochemical and behavioral parallels in aging and hypoxia. Chapter in: *The Aging Brain: Cellular and Molecular Mechanisms of Aging in the Nervous System*, eds. Giacobini, E., Filogamo, G., Giacobini, G., and Veradakis, A., Raven Press, New York, pp. 107-122.

Gibson, G. E. and Peterson, C. (1987). Calcium and the aging nervous system. *Neurobiol. Aging* **8**: 329-343.

Gibson, G., Peterson, C. and Freeman, G. (1987). Alterations in neurotransmitter metabolism and calcium homeostasis during aging and Alzheimer's disease. Chapter in: *Molecular Neuropathology of Aging (Banbury Report 27)*, eds. Davies, P. and Finch, C. E., Cold Springs Harbor Lab., pp. 85-106.

Giorgi, O., Calderini, G., Toffano, G. and Biggio, G. (1987). D-1 dopamine receptors labeled with [^{3}H]SCH-23390: decrease in the striatum of aged rats. *Neurobiol. Aging* **8**: 51-54.

Gonzales, R. A., Brown, L. M., Jones, T. W., Trent, R. D., Westbrook, S. L. and Leslie, S. W. (1991) N-Methyl-D-aspartate mediated responses decrease with age in Fischer 344 rat brain. *Neurobiol. Aging* **12**: 219-225.

Govoni, S., Rius, R. A., Battaini, M. S., Magnoni, M. S., Lucchi, L. and Trabucchi, M. (1988). The central dopaminergic system: susceptibility to risk factors for accelerated aging. *Gerontology* **34**: 29-34.

Gozlan, H., Daval, G., Verge, D., Spampinato, V., Fattaccini, C. M., Gallissot, M. C., El Mestikawy, S. and Hamon, M. (1990). Aging associated changes in serotonergic and dopaminergic pre- and postsynaptic neurochemical markers in the rat brain. *Neurobiol. Aging* **11**: 437-449.

Greenberg, L. H. and Weiss, B. (1979). Ability of aged rats to alter beta adrenergic receptors of brain in response to repeated administration of reserpine and desmethylimipramine. *J. Pharmacol. Exp. Therap.* **211**: 309-316.

Greenwood, C. E. and Cinader, B. (1991) Age-related decline in striatal D_2-dopamine receptors is subject to 'economic correction'. *Gerontology* **37**: 244-253.

Greenwood, C. E., Tatton, W. G., Seniuk, N. A. and Biddle, F. E. (1991). Increased dopamine synthesis in aging substantia nigra neurons. *Neurobiol. Aging* **12**: 557-565.

Henry, J. M. and Roth, G. S. (1984). Effect of aging on recovery of striatal dopamine receptors following N-ethoxy-carbonyl 2-ethoxy-1,2 dihydroquinoline (EEDQ) blockage. *Life Sci.* **35**: 899-904.

Henry, J. M., Filburn, C. R., Joseph, J. A. and Roth, G. S. (1986). Effect of aging on striatal dopamine receptor subtypes in Wistar rats. *Neurobiol. Aging* **7**: 357-361.

Hirschhorn, I. D., Makman, M. H. and Gardner, E. L. (1980). Changes in guanine nucleotide sensitive and insensitive ^{3}H-ADTN binding in striatum following substantia nigra lesions. *Eur. J. Pharmacol.* **62**: 123-124.

Hirschhorn, I. D., Makman, M. H. and Sharpless, N. S. (1982). Dopamine receptor sensitivity following nigrostriatal lesion in the aged rat. *Brain Res.* **234**: 357-368.

Horvath, T. B., and Davis, K. L. (1990) Central nervous system disorders in aging. Chapter in: *Handbook of the Biology of Aging*, eds. Schneider, E. L. and Rowe, J. H., Third Edition, Academic Press, New York, pp. 306-329.

Hyttel, J. M. (1987). Age related decrease in the density of dopamine D1 and D2 receptors in corpus striatum of rats. *Pharmacol. Toxicol.* **61**: 126-129.

Inglefield, J. R. and Richfield, E. K. (1992). Preservation of the density of dopamine uptake complex in aging Fischer 344 rat brain. *Neurobiol. Aging* **13**: 383-391.

Joseph, J. A., Berger, R. E., Engel, B. T. and Roth, G. S. (1978). Age related changes in the neostriatum: a behavioral and biochemical analysis. *J. Gerontol.* **33**: 643-649.

Joyce, J. N., Loeschen, S. K., Sapp, D. W. and Marshall, J. F. (1986). Age-related regional loss of caudate-putamen dopamine receptors revealed by quantitative autoradiography. *Brain Res.* **378**: 158-163.

Kalaria, R. N. and Andorn, A. C. (1992). Adrenergic receptors in aging and Alzheimer's disease: decreased α_2-receptors demonstrated by [^{3}H]p-aminoclonidine binding in prefrontal cortex. *Neurobiol. Aging* **12**: 131-136.

Katz, I. R., Smith, D. and Makman, M. H. (1983). Forskolin stimulates the conversion of tyrosine to dopamine in catecholaminergic neural tissue. *Brain Res.* **264**: 173-177.

Kish, S. J., Shannak, K., Rajput, A., Deck, J. H. N. and Hornykiewicz, O. (1992). Aging produces a specific pattern of striatal dopamine loss: implications for the etiology of idiopathic Parkinson's disease. *J. Neurochem.* **58**: 642-648.

Kurian, P., Narang, N. and Crews, F. T. (1992). Decreassed carbachol-stimulated inositol 1,3,4,5-tetrakisphosphate formation in senescent rat cerebral cortical slices. *Neurobiol. Aging* **13**: 521-526.

Lai, H., Bowden, D. M. and Horita, A. (1987). Age-related decreases in dopamine receptors in the caudate nucleus and putamen of the rhesus monkey (*Macaca mulatta*). *Neurobiol. Aging* **8**: 45-49.

Lakatta, E. G. (1990). Heart and circulation. Chapter in: *Handbook of the Biology of Aging*, eds. Schneider, E. L., and Rowe, J. W., Third Edition, Academic Press, New York, pp. 181-216.

Landfield, P. W. and Pitler, T. A. (1984). Prolonged Ca^{2+}-dependent afterhyperpolarizations in hippocampal neurons of aged rats. *Science* **226**: 1089-1092.

Laping, N. J., Dluzen, D. E. and Ramirez, V. D. (1990). Aging alters opiate inhibition of potassium (K^+)-stimulated dopamine release from the corpus striatum of male rats. *Neurobiol. Aging* **11**: 395-399.

Leprohon-Greenwood, C. E. and Cinader, B. (1987). Variations in age-related decline in striatal D_2-dopamine receptors in a variety of mouse strains. *Mech. Ageing Dev.* **38**: 199-206.

Levin, P., Janda, J. K., Joseph, J. A., Ingram, D. K. and Roth, G. S. (1981). Dietary restriction retards the age associated loss of rat striatal dopaminergic receptors. *Science* **214**: 561-562.

Li, P. P., Vecil, G. G., Green, M. A. and Marsh, J. J. (1992). Inositol 1,4,5-trisphosphate receptor in developing and senescent rat cerebellum. *Neurobiol. Aging* **13**: 89-92.

Lledo, P. M., Homburger, V., Bockaert, J. and Vincent, J.-D. (1992). Differential G protein-mediated coupling of D_2 dopamine receptors to K^+ and Ca^{2+} currents in rat anterior pituitary cells. *Neuron* **8**: 455-463.

Makman, M. H., Ahn, H. S., Thal, L. J., Dvorkin, B., Horowitz, S. G., Sharpless, N. S. and Rosenfeld, M. (1978). Biogenic amine-stimulated adenylate cyclase and spiroperidol-binding sites in rabbit brain: evidence for selective loss of receptors with aging. Chapter in: *Parkinson's Disease – II Aging and Neuroendocrine Relationships (Ad, Exp. Med. Biol., vol. 113)*, eds. Finch, C. E., Potter., D. E. and Kenney, A. D., Plenum Press, New York, 1978, pp. 211-230.

Makman, M. H., Ahn, H. S., Thal, L. J., Sharpless, N. S., Dvorkin, B., Horowitz, S. G. and Rosenfeld, M. (1979). Aging and monoamine receptors in brain. *Federation Proc.* **38**: 1922-1926.

Makman, M. H., Ahn, H. S., Thal, L. J., Sharpless, N. S., Dvorkin, B., Horowitz, S. G. and Rosenfeld, M. (1980a). Evidence for selective loss of brain dopamine- and histamine-stimulated adenylate cyclase activities in rabbits with aging. *Brain Res.* **192**: 177-183.

Makman, M. H., Dvorkin, B. and Klein, P. N. (1982). Sodium ion modulates D_2 receptor characteristics of dopamine agonist and antagonist binding sites in striatum and retina. *Proc. Nat. Acad. Sci. U.S.A.* **79**: 4212-4216.

Makman, M. H., Gardner, E. L., Thal, L. J., Hirschhorn, I. D., Seeger, T. F. and Bhargava, G. (1980b). Central monoamine receptor systems: influence of aging, lesion and drug treatment. Chapter in: *Neural Regulatory Mechanisms During Aging*, eds., Adelman, R. C., Roberts, J., Baker, G. T., Baskin, S. I. and Cristofalo, V. J., Liss, New York, pp. 91-127.

Makman, M. H., O'Connell, M. E., Hirschhorn, I. D., Cubells, J. and Thal, L. J. (1984). Receptor and transmitter interactions of monoamines and neuropeptides: neuroendocrine influences and age-related changes. Chapter in: *Altered Endocrine Status During Aging*, eds., Cristofalo, V. J., Baker, G. T., Adelman, R. C., and Roberts, J., Liss, New York, pp. 35-55.

Marshall, J. F. and Berrios, N. (1979). Movement disorders of aged rats: reversal by dopamine receptor stimulation. *Science* **206**: 447-449.

Marshall, J. F. and Rosenstein, A. J. (1990). Age-related decline in rat striatal dopamine metabolism is regionally homogeneous. *Neurobiol. Aging* **11**: 131-137.

Massie, H. R., Aiello, V. R. and DeWolfe, L. K. (1989). Calcium and calmodulin changes with ageing in C57BL/6J mice. *Gerontology* **35**: 100-105.

McKenzie, F. R. and Milligan, G. (1991). Cholera toxin impairment of opioid-mediated inhibition of adenylate cyclase in neuroblastoma × glioma hybrid cells is due to a toxin-induced decrease in opioid receptor levels. *Biochem. J.* **275**: 175-181.

Michaelis, M. L., Foster, C. T. and Jayawickreme, C. (1992). Regulation of calcium levels in brain tissue from adult and aged rats. *Mech. Ageing Dev.* **62**: 291-306.

Mishra, R. K., Gardner, E. L., Katzman, R. and Makman, M, H. (1974). Enhancement of dopamine-stimulated adenylate cyclase activity in rat caudate after lesions in substantia nigra: evidence for denervation supersensitivity. *Proc. Nat. Acad. Sci. U.S.A.* **71**: 3883-3887.

Morelli, M., Mennini, T., Cagnotto, A., Toffano, G. and Chiara, G. (1990). Quantitative autoradiographical analysis of the age-related modulation of central dopamine D1 and D2 receptors. *Neurosci.* **36**: 403-410.

Morgan, D. G. and Finch, C. E. (1988). Dopaminergic changes in the basal ganglia: a generalized phenomenon of aging mammals. *Ann. New York Acad. Sci.* **515**: 145-160.

Morgan, D. G. and May, P. C. (1990) Age-related changes in synaptic neurochemistry. Chapter in: *Handbook of the Biology of Aging*, eds., Schneider, E. L. and Rowe, J. W., Third Edition, Academic Press, New York, pp. 219-254.

Murray, A. M., and Waddington, J. L. (1991) Age-related changes in the regulation of behavior by D-1:D-2 dopamine receptor interactions. *Neurobiol. Aging* **12**: 431-435.

Narayanan, N. and Derby, J. (1982). Alterations in the properties of beta-adrenergic receptors of myocardial membranes in aging. Impairments of agonist-receptor interactions and guanine nucleotide regulation accompany diminished catecholamine-responsiveness of adenylate cyclase. *Mech. Ageing Dev.* **19**: 127-139.

O'Boyle, K. M. and Waddington, J. L. (1984). Loss of rat striatal dopamine receptors with aging is selective for the D-2 but not the D-1 sites. Association with increased non-specific binding of the D-1 ligand $\pm$ ^{3}H-piflutixol. *Eur. J. Pharmacol.* **105**: 171-174.

O'Connor, S. W., Scarpace, P. J. and Abrass, I. B. (1981). Age-associated decrease of adenylate cyclase activity in rat myocardium. *Mech. Aging Dev.* **16**: 91-95.

Okamoto, T., Murayama, Y., Hayashi, Y., Ingaki, M., Ogata, E. and Nishimoto, I. (1991). Identification of a G_s activator region of the beta-adrenergic receptor that is autoregulated via protein kinase A-dependent phosphorylation. *Cell* **67**: 723-730.

Osterburg, H. H., Donahue, H. G., Severson, J. A. and Finch, C. E. (1981). Catecholamine levels and turnover during aging in brain regions of C57BL/6J mice. *Brain Res.* **224**: 337-352.

Porceddu, M. L., DeMontis, G., Pepitoni, S., Toffano, G. and Biggio, G. (1990). Failure of dark adaptation to upregulate D-1 dopamine receptors in retina of senescent rats. *Neurobiol. Aging* **11**: 105-109.

Puri, S. K. and Volicer, L. (1977). Effect of aging on cyclic AMP levels and adenylate cyclase and phosphodiesterase activities in the rat corpus striatum. *Mech. Ageing Dev.* **6**: 53-58.

Randall, P. K., Severson, J. A. and Finch, C. E. (1981). Aging and the regulation of striatal dopaminergic mechanisms in mice. *J. Pharmacol. Exp. Therap.* **219**: 695-700.

Rinne, J., Lonnberg, P. and Marjamski, P. (1990). Age-dependent decline in human dopamine D1 and D2 receptors. *Brain Res.* **508**: 349-352.

Rossi, G. L., Bestetti, G. E. and Reymond, M. J. (1992). Tuberoinfundibular dopaminergic neurons and lactotropes in young and old female rats. *Neurobiol. Aging* **13**: 275-281.

Roth, G. S. (1982). Altered mechanisms of opiate and dopaminergic action during aging. Chapter in: *The Aging Brain: Cellular and Molecular Mechanisms of Aging in the Nervous System*, eds., Giacobini, E., Filogamo, G., Giacobini, G. and Veradakis, A., Raven Press, New York, pp. 203-209.

Roth, G. S. and Josephs, J. A. (1988). Peculiarities of the effects of hormones and transmitters during aging: modulation of changes in dopaminergic action. *Gerontology* **34**: 22-28.

Scarpace, P. J. (1990). Forskolin activation of adenylate cyclase in rat myocardium with age: effects of guanine nucleotide analogues. *Mech. Aging Dev.* **52**: 169-178.

Schmidt, M. J. and Thornberry, J. F. (1978). Cyclic AMP and cyclic GMP accumulation *in vitro* in brain regions of young and old rats. *Brain Res.* **139**: 169-177.

Severson, J. A. and Finch, C. E. (1980). Reduced dopaminergic binding during aging in the rodent striatum. *Brain Res.* **192**: 147-162.

Severson, J. A. and Randall, P. K. (1985) D-2 dopamine receptors in aging mouse striatum: determination of high and low affinity agonist binding sites. *J. Pharmacol. Exp. Therap.* **233**: 361-368.

Severson, J. A., Marcusson, J., Winblad, B. and Finch, C. E. (1982). Age related changes in dopaminergic binding sites in human basal ganglia. *J. Neurochem.* **39**: 1623-1631.

Severson, J. A., Osterburg, H. H. and Finch, C. E. (1981). Aging and haloperidol-induced dopamine turnover in the nigro-striatal pathway of C57BL/6J mice. *Neurobiol. Aging* **2**: 193-197.

Sidhu, A., Sullivan, M., Kohout, T., Balen, P. and Fishman, P. H. (1991). D_1 dopamine receptors can interact with both stimulatory and inhibitory guanine nucleotide binding proteins. *J. Neurochem.* **57**: 1445-1451.

Sims, N. R., Bowen, D. M., and Davison, A. N. (1982) Acetycholine synthesis and glucose metabolism in aging and dementia. Chapter in: *The Aging Brain: Cellular and Molecular Mechanisms of Aging in the Nervous System*, eds., Giacobini, E., Filogamo, G., Giacobini, G. and Veradakis, A., Raven Press, New York, pp. 153-160.

Tatton, W. G., Greenwood, C. E., Verrier, M. C., Holland, D. P., Kwan, M. M. and Biddle, F. E. (1991). Different rates of age-related loss for four murine monoaminergic neuronal populations. *Neurobiol. Aging* **12**: 543-556.

Thal, L. J., Horowitz, S. G., Dvorkin, B. and Makman, M. H. (1980). Evidence for loss of brain [^{3}H]spiroperidol and [^{3}H]ADTN binding sites in rabbit brain with aging. *Brain Res.* **192**: 185-194.

Timiras, P. S., Hudson, D. B. and Miller, C. (1982) Developing and aging brain serotonergic systems. Chapter in: *The Aging Brain: Cellular and Molecular Mechanisms of Aging in the Nervous System*, eds., Giacobini, E., Filogamo, G., Giacobini, G., and Veradakis, A., Raven Press, New York, pp. 173-184.

Tol, H. H. M., Wu, C. M., Guan, H.-C., Ohara, K., Bunzow, J. R., Civelli, O., Kennedy, J., Seeman, P., Niznik, H. B. and Jovanovic, V. (1992). Multiple dopamine D4 receptor variants in the human population. *Nature* **358**: 149-152.

Trabucchi, M., Spano, P. F., Govoni, S., Riccardi, F., and Bosio, A. (1982) Dopaminergic function during aging in rat brain. Chapter in: *The Aging Brain: Cellular and Molecular Mechanisms of Aging in the Nervous System*, eds., Giacobini, E., Filogamo, G., Giacobini, G. and Veradakis, A., Raven Press, New York, pp. 195-201.

Undies, A. S. and Friedman, E. (1992). Age-induced decrease in dopaminergic-stimulated phosphoinositide metabolism in rat brain. *Neurobiol. Aging* **13**: 505-511.

Van Laijtelaar, M. G. P. A., Tonnaer, J. A. D. M. and Steinbusch, H. W. M. (1992). Aging and the serotonergic system in the rat forebrain: an immunocytochemical and neurochemical study. *Neurobiol. Aging* **13**: 201-216.

Walford, R. L. (1990). The major histocompatibility complex and aging in mammals. *UCLA Symposia on Molecular and Cellular Biology*, New Series, 123: 31-41. Chapter in: *Molecular Biology of Aging*, eds., Finch, C. E. and Johnson, R. E., Wiley-Liss, New York, 1990.

Weiland, N. G., Cohen, I. R. and Wise, P. M, (1989). Age-associated alterations in catecholamine concentrations, neuronal activity, and α_1 receptor densities in female rats. *Neurobiol. Aging* **10**: 323-329.

Wise, P. M., Cohen, I. R. and Weiland, N. G. (1987). Hypothalamic monoamine function during aging: its role in the onset of reproductive infertility. Chapter in: *Molecular Neuropathology of Aging (Banbury Report 27)*, eds., Davies, P. and Finch, C. E., Cold Springs Harbor Lab., pp. 159-168.

Wolf, M. E., LeWitt, P. A., Bannon, M. J., Dragovic, L. J. and Kapatos, G. (1991). Effect of aging on tyrosine hydroxylase protein content and the relative number of dopamine nerve terminals in human caudate. *J. Neurochem.* **65**: 1191-1200.

Yamagami, K., Joseph, J. A. and Roth, G. S. (1992). Muscarinic receptor concentrations and dopamine release in aged rat striata. *Neurobiol. Aging* **13**: 51-56.

Altered Calcium Homeostasis During Aging of the Brain: Cellular Mechanisms Involved and Possible Consequences

JORGINA SATRÚSTEGUI, ALBERTO MARTÍNEZ-SERRANO, PABLO BLANCO, MARTÍN VILLALBA, PAULINO GÓMEZ PUERTAS and ELENA BOGONEZ

Departamento de Biología Molecular (CSIC-UAM), Universidad Autónoma, Canto Blanco, 28049 Madrid, Spain

Introduction

Calcium is an important second messenger involved in nerve cell function. At the nerve terminal, calcium ions trigger the onset of exocytosis, and therefore the fusion of synaptic vehicles and plasma membranes. Calcium levels also regulate important controlling elements of neuronal activity such as protein kinases and phosphatases. These regulators may act on proteins involved in energy metabolism, in neurotransmitter metabolism, on proteins that regulate the excitability of the plasma membrane such as ion channels, and on proteins involved in the organization of the cytoskeleton and its interaction with synaptic vesicles and other organelles (Kennedy, 1989).

In order to perform this role, the free calcium concentration of the cytosol, $[Ca^{2+}]_i$, must be finely regulated. At the nerve terminal, calcium entry from the external medium proceeds mainly via voltage-gated calcium channels (VGCC) and calcium normalization involves extrusion across the plasma membrane (through an electrogenic Na^+/Ca^{2+} exchanger and a Ca^{2+}-dependent ATPase) and sequestration in internal organelles (mitochondria and endoplasmic reticulum, ER) ((Blaustein, 1988).

Voltage-gated calcium channels

The first evidence that calcium homeostasis was altered during aging came from the work of Peterson and Gibson (1983) who found a pronounced decrease in calcium uptake in synaptosomes derived from old rats. These and other authors had found that rat and mouse aging was associated with a reduction in acetylcholine synthesis and release which preceded the loss of cholinergic markers (Gibson and Peterson, 1981; Gibson *et al.*, 1981; Meyer *et al.*, 1984; Pedata *et al.*, 1983). It was thus possible that the reduction in acetylcholine release could be related to a reduced calcium entry via voltage-gated calcium channels, and hence to a reduced availability of calcium for exocitosis (calcium-cholinergic hypothesis). This hypothesis led us to analyze whether $^{45}Ca^{2+}$ entry via VGCC was responsible for the defect in calcium accumulation in synapsotomes from old rats.

To this end, we defined conditions under which other calcium influx pathways except the voltage-gated channels were canceled out and then studied the rate of calcium influx into the nerve terminals as a function of the membrane potential obtained at different depolarizing conditions. The calcium influx rates found followed the Boltzman equation that defines the calcium inflow at any given membrane potential as a function of the maximum inflow through open calcium channels and the midpoint voltage for channel activation. Our results indicated that there was no change in the midpoint voltage and a modest but significant (20%) decrease in calcium inflow through the open calcium channels (Martínez *et al.*, 1987). This decrease was more pronounced when the calcium concentration of the external medium was reduced to below millimolar (Martínez-Serrano *et al.*, 1989). It is unlikely that this defect is due to a reduction in the number of VGCC during aging since Battaini *et al.* (1985) and Dooley *et al.* (1988) have found increased numbers or stability of L and N types of VGCC binding sites in old rats.

Neurons have various types of calcium channels, the so-called L, N and T types, which have different electrophysiological properties (Nowycky *et al.*, 1985). Due to their small size (about 0.5 micron), synaptosomes are not adequate for electrophysiological studies and therefore synaptosomal calcium channels are still unresolved. However, Nachshen together with Suszkiw and coworkers have been able to define some kind of channel diversity in synaptosomes in terms of antagonist sensitivity and inactivation kinetics with the use of calcium flux experiments with a high time resolution (Nachshen, 1985; Suszkiw *et al.*, 1986; 1987; 1989). Thus, synaptosomal VGCC may be different from the classical L or N types (Suszkiw *et al.*, 1989), but possibly similar to type T (Kostyuk, 1989).

To gain some understanding of the type of synaptosomal calcium channels affected by aging, the inactivation of $^{45}Ca^{2+}$ influx via VGCC was studied in rat brain synaptosomes. In the course of depolarization, the instantaneous (2 sec) rate of calcium influx decreases markedly with the length of the depolarization pulse, and a steady state is attained at around 5 sec. This defines an inactivating component and a non-inactivating component which is still present after 20 sec depolarization. Inactivation was slower with aging; the half time of inactivation was 0.7 sec in 3-month-old rats and 0.9 sec in 24-month-old rats. These differences are even larger when inactivation is slowed down by reducing the calcium concentration to 50 μM during the experiment. The inactivating component amounts now to only 35% of the total initial rate and its half time of inactivation goes up to 1.7 sec. Strikingly, under these conditions the inactivating component disappears in old rats. Moreover, the non-inactivating component is also very much reduced (Martínez-Serrano *et al.*, 1989).

Taken together, these results indicate that the activity of synaptosomal calcium channels decreases with age, inactivating and non-inactivating components being both affected, and the onset of this defect, at the age of 12 months, matches very closely the time at which the defect in acetylcholine release appears.

It is interesting to note that Reynolds and Carlen (1989) have also found a significant depression of a high-threshold, slowly-inactivating L-type calcium current in hippocampal dentate gyrus from old rats. These authors have obtained evidence suggesting a substantial calcium-dependent inactivation of VGCC during aging. The results of Applegate and Landfield also suggest an impaired inactivation of presynaptic calcium currents in hippocampus from old rats (Applegate and Landfield, 1988; Landfield, 1988). It is not possible to draw a clear relationship between individual calcium currents as detected in these studies and the components of $^{45}Ca^{2+}$ influx that we have investigated in synaptosomes. Therefore, at present it is still unknown whether the different calcium currents and $^{45}Ca^{2+}$ influx pathways affected by aging are the same or different entities. However, in view of the stability of VGCC numbers (Dooley *et al.*, 1988) and the similarities in inactivation defects observed in old age, it is conceivable that these arise from a common cause, perhaps related to cell calcium homeostasis, as discussed below.

Cytosolic free calcium

The cytosolic free calcium concentration, $[Ca^{2+}]_i$, is the key variable governing the intracellular action of calcium. We have examined the cytosolic free calcium levels in synaptosomes and their changes with aging with the use of fluorescent calcium indicators. Contrary to initial predictions, $[Ca^{2+}]_i$ levels observed under depolarizing conditions were higher rather than lower in old rats as compared to adults. In addition, the same was true under resting conditions (Martínez *et al.*, 1989).

This result was surprising and therefore we have repeated $[Ca^{2+}]_i$ determinations with different methods and with different groups of rats from our colony. The methods have relied on the use of various entrapped fluorescent indicators (quin2, fura2, fluo3) that differ in their spectral characteristics and calcium binding constants (Minta *et al.*, 1989). We would like to point out that we have also employed a method that does not require the introduction of calcium indicators into the cytosol, namely the null point method. Both with this and the other methods, we have consistently observed increased $[Ca^{2+}]_i$ levels in synaptosomes derived from old rats under depolarization, even though the extent of this increase varies with different sets of rats. The same is true for $[Ca^{2+}]_i$ levels at rest. The reasons for this variability are not yet fully understood.

The increase in synaptosomal $[Ca^{2+}]_i$ with age agrees with the findings of Landfield and coworkers who concluded on the basis of electrophysiological experiments that $[Ca^{2+}]_i$ levels in the hippocampus were higher in old rats (Landfield and Pitler, 1984; Kerr *et al.*, 1989). On the other hand, the variability in the size of the increase explains why other authors have failed to detect it (Farrar *et al.*, 1989; Giovanelli and Pepeu, 1989).

Coming back to the initial calcium-cholinergic hypothesis, it is evident that these results do not support it, at least in its present terms. First, $[Ca^{2+}]_i$ are higher rather than lower at depolarization, a factor that would enhance rather than inhibit neurotransmitter release. Second, Meyer *et al.* (1986) have found that after treatment with the calcium ionophore A23187 to trigger acetylcholine release under conditions that would override permeability barriers at the plasma membrane, the age-dependent differences in acetylcholine release persist, indicating that the defect is possibly not due to reduced $[Ca^{2+}]_i$, but to a desensitization or decreased secretory response to calcium ions.

On the other hand, this change in cytosolic free calcium levels may indicate that the systems that govern calcium homeostasis are altered in aging, and this may have important physiopathological consequences. Calcium controls, either by itself or through interaction with calcium binding proteins, the activity of calcium-dependent protein kinases and phosphatases, phospholipases, the assembly and disassembly of cytoskeletal proteins, and these processes are important in the control of cell function and structure. A long-lasting increase in cytosolic calcium is believed to be a critical and non-reversible step leading to cell death in many models of neuronal degeneration, especially those involving excitotoxicity of glutamate (Choi, 1987; Hahn *et al.*, 1989; Boobis *et al.*, 1990). Within this framework, an altered calcium homeostasis during aging may become an age-dependent risk factor for neuronal degeneration and eventually in the pathogenesis of Alzheimer's disease.

The molecular mechanisms responsible for the altered calcium homeostasis in synaptosomes during aging are yet unknown. There are some indications that defects in calcium extrusion systems and calcium binding to the cytosol may be involved. Thus, Michaelis *et al.* (1984) have found that the activity of the plasma membrane Na^+/Ca^{2+} exchanger and Ca^{2+}-ATPase decreased during aging. Results from Christakos's group indicate that there is a specific reduction in calbindin-D_{28K}-gene expression in particular regions of rat, mouse and human brain during aging (Iacopino and Christakos, 1990; Iacopino *et al.*, 1990). Moreover, we have obtained evidence indicating that the calcium binding capacity of the cytosolic compartment in synaptosomes decreases with age, and that calcium extrusion through the Na^+/Ca^{2+} exchanger and, specially, the Ca^{2+}-ATPase, is severely reduced in old rats (Martínez-Serrano *et al.*, 1992).

Defects in calcium accumulation in intracellular organelles may also be involved in altered calcium homeostasis. We have not found any changes in caffeine-sensitive E.R.-type calcium stores (Martínez-Serrano and Satrústegui, 1989) in old animals (Martínez-Serrano, 1992). However, it has become clear that calcium accumulation in mitochondria is severely impaired in old animals.

Mitochondria

Evidence for a role of mitochondria in the decreased calcium uptake in synaptosomes was obtained from experiments in which calcium-loaded synaptosomes incubated in a high-K^+ medium were treated with an uncoupler (FCCP), whereupon a rapid release of calcium was observed. The calcium released upon FCCP treatment is thought to reflect the mitochondrial calcium pool, and represents around 6.9 nmoles/mg protein 3-month-old rats and only 3.7 nmoles/mg protein 24-month-old rats. By dividing mitochondrial (FCCP-releaseable) by extramitochondrial (total minus FCCP-releaseable) calcium, it was observed that the quotient decreased from 0.62 to 0.39 at 3 and 24 months of age, respectively (Vitorica and Satrústegui, 1986a).

It is now well established that there is a specific impairment in the calcium uptake system which is responsible for this mitochondrial defect (Vitorica and Satrústegui, 1986a, b; Leslie *et al.*, 1985; Peterson *et al.*, 1985). The energy transducing ability of the so-called "free" mitochondrial preparation, which includes both the synaptosomal and cell body mitochondria, is not changed with aging when succinate is used as a respiratory source (Vitorica *et al.*, 1985), and therefore it allows us to determine differences in calcium transport under conditions of controlled driving forces. By using these conditions, it was found that the activity of the calcium uniporter of brain mitochondria decreases with aging over a range of calcium concentrations. A Hill plot of the results indicated that Hill numbers decreased whereas $S_{0.5}$ showed a tendency to increase with age from around 1.1 μM to 2.1 μM in 3- and 24-month-old rats, respectively (Vitorica and Satrústegui, 1986a; Satrústegui *et al.*, 1990). Moreover, these changes are probably not due to modifications in the lipid fluidity of the inner mitochondrial membrane, since even though this was reduced in "free" mitochondria (a result reminiscent to that found in mitochondria from other sources) (Vorbeck *et al.*, 1982), it was not changed in intrasynaptosomal mitochondria from old rats, where the impairment of the uniporter activity is clearly present (Vitorica and Satrústegui, 1986a). In addition to this defect, it was observed that the calcium buffering power of the mitochondrial matrix increased with aging, i.e., at equivalent calcium loads, a smaller fraction of that is free in old than in adult animals (Vitorica and Satrústegui, 1986b).

It is now known that the calcium accumulated in mitochondria is not merely stored there, but acts as a regulator of mitochondrial dehydrogenases (McCormick and Denton, 1986; Hansford, 1985). Since brain mitochondria derived from old animals take up less calcium than that derived from adults, and a smaller fraction of that is free in the matrix, this could provide conditions where the regulation by calcium of mitochondrial enzymes is impaired.

This possibility has been examined in the case of pyruvate dehydrogenase. Part of the metabolic control of this enzyme is achieved by a phosphorylation/dephosphorylation cycle catalyzed by kinase and a phosphatase that act on the alpha subunit of the PDH complex. The phosphoenzyme is the catalytically inactive form. Denton *et al.* (1972) discovered that the alpha PDH phosphatase activity was enhanced by micromolar concentrations of calcium, the net effect being an increase in the V_{max} of the PDH complex. We have studied the changes in the phosphorylation state of a 42 KD phosphoprotein band corresponding to alpha PDH in free mitochondria and synaptosomes from 3- and 24-month-old animals. Our results indicate that the dephosphorylation rate of the 42 KD band under conditions of limited calcium entry in mitochondria is reduced in old animals (Bogonez *et al.*, 1988; Satrústegui *et al.*, 1990).

These results suggest that the calcium-dependent activation of pyruvate dehydrogenase is reduced during aging. Pyruvate dehydrogenase is one among a number of factors that can regulate acetylcholine synthesis. *In vivo* acetylcholine synthesis from ^{14}C-glucose decreases with aging (Gibson *et al.*, 1981) and this reduction has been associated with a loss of psychomotor performance of the old animals (Gibson and Peterson, 1982). The finding of a decreased dephosphorylation of the 42 KD band in response to calcium in mitochondria derived from old animals suggests that variations in PDH activation brought about by calcium in response to stimulation could be associated with this defect. This allows a new formulation of the calcium-cholinergic hypothesis whereby the altered calcium uptake in mitochondria during stimulation of nerve terminals may be involved in reduced acetylcholine synthesis and release.

Conclusion

In sum, present evidence suggests that some of the systems that govern calcium homeostasis are altered during aging and this may have important physiopathological consequences. Increased $[Ca^{2+}]_i$, due perhaps to a reduced calcium buffering power in the cytosol and decreased calcium extrusion through plasma membrane Ca^{2+}-ATPase, may be involved in the decreased activity of voltage-gated calcium channels. The decreased activity of the calcium uniporter of mitochondria could be associated with an impaired calcium-dependent activation of pyruvate dehydrogenase and acetylcholine synthesis. These combined effects on cell calcium homeostasis may constitute an age-dependent risk factor for neuronal degeneration.

Acknowledgements

Supported by grants from CICYT (PB86-0520, PB89-0159), from Boheringer Ingelheim, S.A. and by an institutional grant from the Fundación Ramón Areces.

References

Applegate, D. M. and Landfield, P. W. (1988). Synaptic vehicle redistribution during hippocampal frequency potentiation and depression in young and aged rats. *J. Neurosci.* **8**: 1096-1111.

Battaini, F., Govoni, S., Rius, R. N. and Trabucchi, M. (1985). Age-dependent increase in [^{3}H] verapamil binding to rat cortical membranes. *Neurosci. Lett.* **61**: 67-71.

Blaustein, M. (1988). Calcium transport and buffering in neurons. *Trends in Neurosci.* **11**: 438-443.

Bogonez, E., Martínez, A., Blanco, P. and Satrústegui, J. (1988). Effects of aging on depolarization dependent dephosphorylation of synaptosomal proteins. *Neurochem. Int.* **13**: S92.

Boobis, A. R., Fawthrop, D. J. and Davis, D. S. (1990). Mechanisms of cell toxicity. *Curr. Opinion in Cell Biol.* **2**: 231-237.

Choi, D. W. (1987). Ionic dependence of glutamate neurotoxicity. *J. Neurosci.* **7**: 369-379.

Denton, R. M., Randle, P. J. and Martin, B. R. (1972). Stimulation by calcium ions of pyruvate dehydrogenase phosphate phosphatase. *Biochem. J.* **128**: 161-163.

Dooley, D. J., Lickert, M., Lupp, A. and Osswald, H. (1988). Distribution of [^{125}I]ω-conotoxin GVIA and [^{3}H] isradipine binding sites in the central nervous system of rats of different ages. *Neurosci. Lett.* **93**: 318-323.

Farrer, R. P., Rezazadeh, S. M., Morris, J. L., Dildy, J. E., Gnau, K. and Leslie, S. W. (1989). Aging does not alter cytosolic calcium levels of cortical synaptosomes in Fischer 344 rats. *Neurosci. Lett.* **100**: 319-325.

Gibson, G. E. and Peterson, C. (1981). Aging decreases oxidative metabolism and the release and synthesis of acetylcholine. *J. Neurochem.* **37**: 978-984.

Gibson, G. E. and Peterson, C. (1982). Biochemical and behavioral parallels in aging and hypoxia. In: *The Aging Brain. Cellular and Molecular Mechanisms of Aging in the Nervous System*, eds., E. Giacobini *et al.*, Raven Press, New York, pp. 107-122.

Gibson, G. E., Peterson, C. and Jenden, D. J. (1981). Brain acetylcholine synthesis declines with senescence. *Science* **213**: 674-676.

Giovanelli, L. and Pepeu, G. (1989). Effect of age on K^+-induced cytosolic Ca^{2+} changes in rat cortical synaptosomes. *J. Neurochem.* **53**: 392-398.

Hahn, J. S., Aizenman, E. and Lipton, S. A. (1988). Central mammalian neurons normally resistant to glutamate toxicity are made sensitive by elevated extracellular Ca^{2+}: Toxicity is blocked by the N-methyl-D-aspartate antagonist MK-801. *Proc. Natl. Acad. Sci. U.S.A.* **85**: 6556-6560.

Hansford, R. G. (1985). Relation between mitochondrial calcium transport and control of energy metabolism. *Rev. Physiol. Biochem. Pharmacol.* **102**: 1-72.

Iacopino, A. M. and Christakos, S. (1990). Specific reduction of calcium-binding protein (28-kilodalton calbindin-D) gene expression in aging and neurodegenerative diseases. *Proc. Natl. Acad. Sci. U.S.A.* **87**: 4078-4082.

Iacopino, A. M., Rhoten, W. B. and Christakos, S. (1990). Calcium binding protein (calbindin-D_{28K}) gene expression in the developing and aging mouse cerebellum. *Mol. Brain Res.* **8**: 283-290.

Kennedy, M. B. (1989). Regulation of neuronal function by calcium. *Trends in Neurosci.* **12**: 417-420.

Kerr, D. S., Campbell, L. W., Hao, S. Y. and Landfield, P. W. (1989). Corticosteroid modulation of hippocampal potentials: Increased effect with aging. *Science* **245**: 1505-1509.

Kostyuk, P. G. (1989). Diversity of calcium channels in cellular membranes. *Neurosci.* **28**: 253-261.

Landfield, P. M. (1988). Hippocampal neurobiological mechanisms of age-related memory dysfunction. *Neurobiol. Aging* **9**: 571-579.

Landfield, P. W. and Pitler, T. A. (1984). Prolonged Ca^{2+}-dependent after hyperpolarizations in hippocampal neurons of aged rats. *Science* **226**: 1089-1092.

Leslie, S. W., Chandler, L. J., Barr, E. M. and Farrar, R. P. (1985). Reduced calcium uptake by rat brain mitochondria and synaptosomes in response to aging. *Brain Res.* **329**: 177-183.

MacCormack, J. G. and Denton, R. M. (1986). Ca^{2+} as a second messenger within mitochondria. *Trends Biochem. Sci.* **11**: 258-262.

Martínez, A., Vitorica, J. and Satrústegui, J. (1988). Cytosolic free calcium levels increase with age in rat brain synaptosomes. *Neurosci. Lett.* **88**: 336-342.

Martínez, A., Vitorica, J., Bogonez, E. and Satrústegui, J. (1987). Differential effects of age on the pathways of calcium influx into nerve terminals. *Brain Res.* **435**: 249-257.

Martínez-Serrano, A. and Satrústegui, J. (1989). Caffeine-sensitive calcium stores in presynaptic nerve endings: A physiological role? *Biochem. Biophys. Res. Commun.* **161**: 965-971.

Martínez-Serrano, A., Bogonez, E., Vitorica, J. and Satrústegui, J. (1989). Reduction of K^+-stimulated $^{45}Ca^{2+}$ influx in synaptosomes with age involves inactivating and noninactivating calcium channels and is correlated with temporal modifications in protein dephosphorylation. *J. Neurochem.* **52**: 576-584.

Martínez-Serrano, A., Blanco, P. and Satrústegui, J. (1992). Calcium binding to the cytosol and calcium extrusion mechanisms in intact synaptosomes and their alterations with aging. *J. Biol. Chem.* **267**: 4672-4679

Meyer, E. M., Crews, F. T., Otero, D. H. and Larsen, K. (1986). Aging decreases the sensitivity of rat cortical synaptosomes to calcium ionophore-induced acetylcholine release. *J. Neurochem.* **47**: 1244-1246.

Meyer, E. M., St. Once, E. and Crews, F. T. (1984). Effects of aging on rat cortical presynaptic cholinergic processes. *Neurobiol. Aging* **5**: 315-317.

Michaelis, M. L., Johe, K. and Kitos, T. E. (1984). Age-dependent alterations in synaptic membrane systems for Ca^{2+} regulation. *Mech. Age Devel.* **25**: 215-225.

Minta, A., Kao, J. P. Y. and Tsien, R. Y. (1989). Fluorescent indicators for cytosolic calcium based on rhodamine and fluorescein chromophores. *J. Biol. Chem.* **264**: 8171-8178.

Nachshen, D. A. (1985). The early time course of potassium-stimulated calcium uptake in presynaptic nerve-terminals isolated from rat brain. *J. Physiol. (London)* **361**: 251-268.

Nowycky, M. D., Fox, A. P. and Tsien, R. W. (1985). Three types of neuronal calcium channels with different calcium agonist sensitivity. *Nature* **316**: 440-443.

Pedata, F., Slavikova, Y., Kotas, A. and Papeu, G. (1983). Acetylcholine release from rat cortical slices during postnatal development and aging. *Neurobiol. Aging* **4**: 31-34.

Peterson, C. and Gibson, G. E. (1983). Aging and 3,4-diaminopyridine alter synaptosomal calcium uptake. *J. Biol. Chem.* **258**: 11482-11486.

Peterson, C., Nicholls, D. G. and Gibson, G. E. (1985). Subsynaptosomal calcium distribution during aging and 3,4-diaminopyridine treatment. *Neurobiol. Aging* **6**: 297-304.

Reynolds, J. N. and Carlen, P. L. (1989). Diminished calcium current in aged hippocampal dentate gyrus granule neurons. *Brain Res.* **479**: 384-390.

Satrústegui, J., Martínez-Serrano, A., Blanco, P. and Bogonez, E. (1990). Influence of aging on the compartmentation of calcium within nerve endings during depolarization and effects on pyruvate dehydrogenase dephosphorylation. In: *Theoretical Basis of Aging Research*, eds., L. Robert and G. Hofecker, Facultas Verlag, Wien, pp. 265-274.

Suszkiw, J. B., Murawsky, M. M. and Fortner, R. C. (1987). Heterogeneity of presynaptic calcium channels revealed by species differences in the sensitivity of synaptosomal $^{45}Ca^{2+}$ entry to ω-conotoxin. *Biochem. Biophys. Res. Commun.* **145**: 1283-1286.

Suszkiw, J. B., Murawsky, M. M. and Shi, M. (1989). Further characterization of phasic calcium influx in rat cerebrocortical synaptosomes: Inferences regarding calcium types in nerve endings. *J. Neurochem.* **52**: 1260-1269.

Suszkiw, J. B., O'Leary, M. E., Murawsky, M. M. and Wang, T. (1986). Presynaptic calcium channels in rat cortical synaptosomes: fast kinetics of phasic calcium influx, channel inactivation, and relationship to nitrendipine receptors. *J. Neurosci.* **6**: 1349-1357.

Vitorica, J. and Satrústegui, J. (1986a). Involvement of mitochondria in the age-dependent decrease in calcium uptake in rat brain synaptosomes. *Brain Res.* **378**: 36-48.

Vitorica, J. and Satrústegui, J. (1986b). The influence of age on the calcium-effflux pathway and matrix calcium buffering power in brain mitochondria. *Biochem. Biophys. Acta* **851**: 209-216.

Vitorica, J., Clark, A., Machado, A. and Satrústegui, J. (1985). Impairment of glutamate uptake and absence of alterations in energy transducing ability in old rat brain mitochondria. *Mech. Ageing Devel.* **29**: 255-266.

Vorbeck, M. L., Martin, A. P., Long, J. W. Jr., Smith, J. M. and Orr, R. R. Jr. (1982). Aging-dependent modification of lipid composition and lipid structural order parameter of hepatic mitochondria. *Arch. Biochem. Biophys.* **217**: 351-361.

Adrenal Glucocorticoids as Modulators of Brain Aging

MICHAEL J. MEANEY, SHARI R. BODNOFF, SEEMA BHATNAGAR, DAJAN O'DONNELL, SHARON A. WELNER and JUDES POIRIER

Aging Research Program, McGill University-Douglas Hospital Research Center, Departments of Psychiatry, Neurology and Neurosurgery, and Experimental Medicine, McGill University, Montreal, Canada

Introduction

Variation in magnitude of cognitive decline in later life is a central feature of human aging. The more severe forms of dementia, such as Alzheimer's disease, clearly define one end of the spectrum. However, among those showing no obvious signs of clinical dementia there are considerable individual differences. Thus, while evidence for learning, memory, and language loss appears in some individuals as early as 50-55 years of age, many people continue to function alertly well into their nineties. These individuals exemplify what Rowe and Kahn (1987) have termed "successful" aging. These dramatic individual differences in CNS aging, usually a nuisance factor in many earlier studies, are becoming a major focus for brain aging research (e.g., Gage *et al.*, 1984, 1986; Gallager *et al.*, 1990; Issa *et al.*, 1990).

This approach to the topic of brain aging differs from that of many research groups where the emphasis is on the identification of factors that are involved in the etiology of specific forms of dementia, such as Alzheimer's disease. One major objective for studies of individual differences in brain aging is to examine the full range of "normal" processes of CNS aging and to understand how these processes differ, in kind or degree, from neuropathological states. In doing so, one can study the entire range of CNS states in later life, including possible determinants of milder forms of neurological and cognitive impairments (e.g. age-associated memory impairments) as well, of course, as individuals in whom there is no evidence for neuropathology or cognitive decline. It is very likely that the prevalence and the impact of these milder forms of neurological/cognitive impairments have been underestimated. Some reports claim that perhaps as many as 90% of all people over 65 years of age suffer measurable memory problems (see Bartus and Dean, 1987). The degree to which these impairments interfere with daily life will very much depend upon the demands placed upon the individual. However, there can be no doubt that in a great many cases the restrictions associated with these impairments do indeed compromise the quality of life. Thus, in addition to discernible cases of clinical dementia, there exists evidence for a substantial health problem associated with CNS aging that involves milder forms of cognitive impairments.

Research focusing on the heterogeneity in CNS aging is absolutely essential. To some extent, there persists a tendency to use the variable of age as if it were a sufficient explanation of functional change (see Rowe and Kahn, 1987). Considering the individual variation in CNS function among aged mammals, it is clear that chronological age alone can explain very little. Instead, research should attempt to identify the specific mechanisms responsible for functional decline, as well as the factors that might explain instances where such decline is absent. If we are able to identify factors that account for variations in CNS aging, the prospects for avoiding or even reversing functional loss become greatly enhanced.

In this research we are making the assumption that functional decline is associated with neurological deficits, such as neuron loss. The emphasis in our studies, then, is to understand the hormonal factors that might account for individual differences in neuron loss and possibly a decline in the capacity of surviving neurons to compensate for such a loss. These studies follow from an hypothesis advanced by Selye concerning the role of stress in age-related dysfunction. Selye (1950) proposed that stress drains the body of "adaptive energy" and therefore accelerates the degeneration associated with aging. The studies reviewed here suggest that in fact it is the stress hormones associated with the organism's adaptational responses to stress that potentiate neuronal dysfunction in later life. However, in addition to focusing on the amount of stress to which an animal is exposed, we must also consider individual differences in the ability to effectively control the secretion of certain stress hormones; this factor may be critical in predicting the occurrence of some forms of age-related neuropathology.

The hypothalamic-pituitary-adrenal (HPA) axis

The HPA response to stress is a basic adaptive mechanism in mammals. Together with the catecholamines, the glucocorticoids secreted by the adrenal cortex account for most of the physiological responses to stimuli that threaten homeostasis. Pituitary-adrenal activity lies under the dominion of CNS control, most notably the secretion of peptidergic releasing factors emanating from the mediobasal hypothalamus. Thus, during stress the increased secretion of corticotropin-releasing hormone (CRH) and co-secretagogues, such as vasopressin (AVP) and oxytocin, into the portal system of the anterior pituitary enhances the synthesis and release of proopiomelanocortin-derived peptides, adrenocorticotropin (ACTH) and β-endorphin (Anton, 1986; Gibbs, 1986; Linton *et al.*, 1985; Nakane *et al.*, 1985; Plotsky, 1987; Rivier and Vale, 1983; Rivier and Plotsky, 1986; Rivier *et al.*, 1982). Elevated ACTH levels, in turn, increase the synthesis and release of adrenal glucocorticoids. The highly catabolic glucocorticoids produce lypolysis, glycogenolysis, and protein catabolism, resulting directly or indirectly (through gluconeogenesis) in increased blood glucose levels (Baxter and Tyrrell, 1987; Munck *et al.*, 1984). These actions assist the organism during stress, in part, by increasing the availability of energy substrates at the expense of existing energy stores and of anabolic processes. Glucocorticoids also suppress immunological responses (Munck *et al.*, 1984), decreasing inflammation when mobility may be essential.

However, prolonged exposure to elevated glucocorticoid levels can present a serious risk, leading to a suppression of anabolic processes, muscle atrophy, decreased sensitivity to insulin and a risk of steroid-induced diabetes, hypertension, hyperlipidemia, hypercholesterolemia, arterial disease, amenorrhea, impotency, and the impairment of growth and tissue repair, as well as immunosuppression (Baxter and Tyrrell, 1987; Munck *et al.*, 1984). Thus, once the stressor is terminated, it is in the animal's best interest to "turn off" the HPA stress response and the efficacy of this process is determined by the ability of the glucocorticoids to inhibit subsequent ACTH release (i.e. glucocorticoid negative feedback).

Circulating glucocorticoids feed back onto the pituitary and specific brain regions to inhibit the secretion of releasing factors from hypothalamic neurons and ACTH from pituitary corticotrophes (Dallman *et al.*, 1987; Jones *et al.*, 1982; Keller-Wood and Dallman, 1984; Plotsky and Vale, 1984; Plotsky *et al.*, 1987; Van Loon and DeSouza, 1987). In addition to these target sites, there is now considerable evidence for the importance of hippocampal inhibition of HPA activity (Dallman *et al.*, 1987; McEwen, 1982). The hippocampus is the major target site in the brain for glucocorticoids and a principal source of negative-feedback inhibition over HPA activity. Hippocampal lesions or ablations are associated with elevated glucocorticoid levels under basal, stress, and post-stress conditions (Feldman and Conforti, 1976, 1980; Fischette *et al.*, 1980; Sapolsky *et al.*, 1984a; Wilson *et al.*, 1980), reduced suppression of ACTH following exogenous glucocorticoid administration (Feldman and Conforti, 1976), and increased hypothalamic CRH and AVP mRNA levels (Herman *et al.*, 1989).

Likewise, there is evidence for the role of the hippocampal corticosteroid receptor systems in mediating negative-feedback inhibition over HPA activity. The hippocampus contains two, distinct receptor sites for corticosterone (the principal glucocorticoid in the rat; Beaumont and Fanestil, 1983; Coirini *et al.*, 1985; Emadian *et al.*, 1986; Funder and Sheppard, 1987; Krozowski and Funder, 1983; Reul and DeKloet, 1985, 1986; Wrange and Yu, 1983). The first (type I receptor) is a mineralocorticoid site, which binds with high affinity to aldosterone, corticosterone, and the synthetic mineralocorticoids, such as RU 26752. The second (type II receptor) is a glucocorticoid site which also binds with high affinity to corticosterone and the synthetic glucocorticoids dexamethasone and RU 28362. There is considerable evidence for the role of the hippocampal glucocorticoid receptor in regulating HPA activity under conditions of elevated plasma glucocorticoid levels. (1) Stress results in a dramatic increase in the hormone-receptor signal (Meaney *et al.*, 1988a; Reul and DeKloet, 1985; Reul *et al.*, 1987). While only about 10-15% of the glucocorticoid receptors are occupied under basal conditions, 75% occupancy accompanies stress (or glucocorticoid injections that mimic steroid levels occurring during stress). (2) Hippocampal implants of the glucocorticoid receptor antagonist, RU 38486, produces elevated levels of plasma ACTH under both basal (Bradbury and Dallman, 1989) and post-stress conditions (Ratka *et al.*, 1989). (3) Decreased hippocampal glucocorticoid receptor density is consistently associated with corticosterone hypersecretion following the termination of stress (McEwen *et al.*, 1986; Meaney *et al.*, 1989a; Sapolsky *et al.*, 1984a,b, 1986a; Sapolsky and Meaney, 1986; Stern and Levine, 1974). In the case of the vasopressin-deficient Brattleboro rat, the hippocampal glucocorticoid receptor deficit is reversed with vasopressin and so long as the treatment is continued, the glucocorticoid receptor levels remain elevated and the animals exhibit normal corticosterone secretion following stress (Sapolsky *et al.*, 1984a). Recently, Dallman's laboratory (see Dallman *et al.*, 1987) has also provided evidence for the importance of the hippocampal mineralocorticoid receptor in the regulation of ACTH. Taken together, these findings suggest that the loss of corticosteroid receptors probably decreases the sensitivity of the hippocampus to circulating glucocorticoids (the signal which initiates negative feedback) which, in turn, dampens negative feedback inhibition, and there ensues an increase in HPA activity and in circulating glucocorticoid levels (see Sapolsky *et al.*, 1986a).

HPA function in the aged rat

Basal levels of plasma ACTH and corticosterone have frequently been reported to be increased with age in the rat (Rapaport *et al.*, 1964; Sencar-Cupovic and Milkovic, 1976; Tang and Philips, 1978; Sapolsky *et al.*, 1983a; Brett *et al.*, 1983; DeKosky *et al.*, 1984; Meaney *et al.*, 1988b, 1991a, 1991b). However, this effect has not always been found (Sonntag *et al.*, 1987), and there is considerable individual variation in HPA function among aged rats (see below). There do not appear to be any major changes in plasma binders for corticosterone with age (Sapolsky, 1983a); however, this topic has not been extensively studied. The clearance rate for corticosterone also appears to be unchanged with age. Thus, changes in measures of total corticosterone likely reflect differences in the magnitude of the free (biologically active) corticoid signal (also see below).

In response to stress, the rat is able to mobilize a 3- to 10-fold increase in plasma corticosterone levels, depending upon the intensity of the stressor. The changes in basal HPA activity have been observed in both male and female rats. However, there is an interesting sex difference in the effects of age on HPA activity during stress. Male rats show little change in plasma corticosterone levels achieved during stress (see Sapolsky, 1987). In contrast, aged female rats show decreased plasma corticosterone levels with stress (Brett *et al.*, 1983; Hess and Reigle, 1970). However, since levels of the principal plasma binder, the estrogen-sensitive corticosterone binding globulin (CBG; Gala and Westphal, 1965), also decrease somewhat with age in females, levels of the free form of the steroid very likely remain constant. In general, it seems that the corticoid signal mobilized during stress is not altered over the course of aging.

In young adult animals, plasma corticosterone levels remain elevated for about 60-120 min following stress. With age, there is a pronounced increase in the duration of the elevated glucocorticoid levels. At 20-26 months of age, plasma corticosterone levels in the adult male remain elevated for as long as 180-360 min following the termination of the stressor (Meaney *et al.*, 1988b; Sapolsky *et al.*, 1983a); even somewhat longer than aged female rats (Meaney *et al.*, 1991a).

Thus, compared with a younger animal, the aged rat shows an impaired ability to terminate an HPA response to stress.

These findings indicate that the corticoid signal in both sexes is elevated with age under basal and post-stress conditions. This increase in HPA activity is likely associated with decreased glucocorticoid negative-feedback inhibition over hypothalamic-pituitary activity. Dilman (1981) reported that there is significantly reduced suppression of HPA function following dexamethasone administration in the aged rat. Moreover, there is a decrease in the suppression of stress-induced HPA activity by exogenous corticosterone treatment in the aged male rat (Sapolsky *et al.*, 1986b). This dampened corticoid inhibition of HPA function corresponds to a loss of brain corticosteroid receptors. In the aged rat there is a loss of both mineralocorticoid and glucocorticoid receptors for corticosterone in the hippocampus (Sapolsky *et al.*, 1983b; Ritger *et al.*, 1984; Meaney *et al.*, 1988b, 1991a, 1991b; Reul *et al.*, 1988), as well as a decrease in the mRNA for the glucocorticoid receptor (Peiffer *et al.*, 1991; van Eckelen, submitted). It is interesting to note that the pattern of negative feedback impairment in the aged rat parallels the effects of hippocampal lesions (see previous section). Thus, the aged rat loses corticosteroid receptors in a brain region that is central for CNS negative feedback control over HPA activity. At this point, it appears that the loss of hippocampal corticosteroid receptors might underlie the decrease in negative feedback control, leading to increased HPA activity under both basal and post-stress conditions.

The HPA axis and brain aging: neuron loss

Hippocampal neuron loss is commonly seen in aged rats (see Coleman and Flood, 1987). In a series of studies, Landfield *et al.* (1978, 1981) demonstrated that the occurrence of hippocampal neuron loss was positively correlated with the increase in HPA activity. They then adrenalectomized rats at mid-life (12 months of age, with low-level corticosterone replacement) and found that these animals showed little or no evidence of hippocampal neuron loss or the spatial memory deficits that are common in later life and closely associated with hippocampal dysfunction. Sapolsky *et al.* (1985) found that young adult rats treated for 3 months with exogenous corticosterone in the upper physiological range (mimicking the elevated basal levels seen in certain old rats) showed profound hippocampal cell loss. Moreover, the pattern of the neuron loss was strikingly similar to that observed in aged animals.

Glucocorticoids are probably not directly responsible for the loss of hippocampal neurons in the aged rat. Rather, the elevated corticosterone levels appear to potentiate neuron loss by rendering hippocampal neurons metabolically vulnerable. The basis for this hypothesis has come from a series of elegant studies by Sapolsky's group (Packan and Sapolsky, 1990; Sapolsky, 1985a, 1985b, 1986; Sapolsky and Pulsinelli, 1985; Sapolsky *et al.*, 1988). These studies are based on the observation that glucocorticoids inhibit glucose uptake by hippocampal neurons (Homer and Sapolsky, 1988). Neurons are notoriously expensive cells for the organism. They have very limited energy storage capacity and a high metabolic rate (Seisjo, 1981). Thus, it is easy to understand how a blockade on glucose uptake might compromise the viability of hippocampal neurons. Not surprisingly, elevated glucocorticoids increase the damage to hippocampal neurons associated with a wide range of insults, including excitotoxins, antimetabolites (i.e., 3-acetylpyridine), oxygen radical generators, and hypoxic-ischemia. These effects can be observed both *in vivo* and *in vitro*, and are not due to any direct interaction between the steroid and the toxins (glucocorticoids do not directly alter the toxicity of the insult). Rather, the corticoids appear to increase the vulnerability of the neurons to the toxins by decreasing the metabolic capacity of the cells to survive the insult. Thus, the ability of elevated glucocorticoid levels to potentiate the damage associated with a wide range of toxins is blocked by supplementary administration of additional energy substrates such as mannose and ketone bodies (Sapolsky, 1986).

The HPA axis and brain aging: short-term effects on hippocampal function

In addition to these long-term effects on neuron survival, exposure to elevated glucocorticoid levels also seems to alter cognitive function in a short-term manner. The fact that many of these effects are reversed following the removal of the enhanced corticoid signal suggests that they are not related to neuron loss. There are several reports (e.g., Starkman *et al.*, 1981; Whelan *et al.*, 1980) of impaired cognitive function associated with elevated glucocorticoid levels of an either endogenous (e.g., Cushing's disease) or exogenous origin (glucocorticoid therapies), and the degree of impaired cognitive function is correlated with cortisol levels (Starkman *et al.*, 1981). Interestingly, these conditions are also associated with evidence (obtained using CT scans) of cerebral atrophy (Benston *et al.*, 1978; Heinz *et al.*, 1977; Okuno *et al.*, 1980). Both the impaired cognitive functioning and the cerebral atrophy are reversed following a decline in glucocorticoid levels. Taken together, these reports indicate that elevated glucocorticoid levels can compromise brain function over a short term of exposure, independent of their effects on neuron loss.

It has been known for some time that glucocorticoids can decrease unit activity in the dorsal hippocampus (Pfaff, Siva and Weiss, 1971). However, the mechanisms underlying these effects are only now becoming clarified. In a series of papers, Joels and DeKloet (1989) and Kerr *et al.* (1989) have demonstrated that in young adult rats glucocorticoids increase both the amplitude and the duration of calcium-dependent slow afterhyperpolarization (AHP) in dorsal hippocampus slice preparations. The effect is mediated by glucocorticoid receptors and the time course is consistent with that of a genomic effect. Such AHPs dampen the neurons' response to subsequent excitatory inputs. Glucocorticoids also decrease the norephinephrine-evoked augmentation of depolarization-induced neuronal activity in Ca_1 neurons. Together, these effects would serve to decrease overall excitability in hippocampal neurons. Kerr *et al.* (1989) demonstrated that the same pattern of effects is apparent in aged rats and is reversed when the animals are adrenalectomized.

Interestingly, Kerr *et al.* (1989) also provided evidence that the increased slow AHP was mediated by an increase in calcium conductance (slow AHPs are related to slow calcium-dependent potassium conductance). The effect on calcium homeostasis is of considerable interest considering the wealth of evidence demonstrating the cytotoxic effects of elevated intracellular calcium. Indeed, there may occur a continuum of glucocorticoid effects. In the early stages, the elevated glucocorticoid signal might be associated with elevated calcium-dependent AHPs, compromising hippocampal function, and continued exposure to elevated glucocorticoid levels might then result in neuron death.

The results of these studies provide clear evidence of short-term effects of glucocorticoids on hippocampal function. These findings also suggest that cognitive processes dependent on hippocampal function would be compromised in the presence of elevated glucocorticoid levels (again, independent of neuron loss). Evidence for such an effect has emerged from experiments using the long-term potentiation model of synaptic plasticity (an electrophysiological model for learning and memory). In one study, Rose and colleagues (G. Rose, pers. comm.) found that LTP induction was increased in adrenalectomized animals and that corticosterone replacement resulted in a dose-dependent decrease in the LTP induction. These data demonstrate that glucocorticoids can impair electrophysiological signal processing in the hippocampus and provide a mechanism for the impaired cognitive function associated with exposure to high corticoid levels.

The HPA axis and brain aging: recovery of function

Partial deafferentation in selected regions of the adult brain results in a sequence of compensatory events involving both the remaining afferent fibers and denervated dendrites, culminating in a reorganization of the circuitry in the denervated area. These events include "sprouting" of the remaining afferent fibers, restoration of spine density and length, and replacement of vacated synaptic contacts. This phenomenon of reactive synaptogenesis has provided one of the most interesting models for the study of the local response to damage in the CNS. One of the best examples of such reactive synaptogenesis occurs in the dentate gyrus of the hippocampus in animals following entorhinal cortex lesions (Lee *et al.*, 1977; Matthews *et al*, 1976; Scheff *et al.*, 1980a). Entorhinal cortex lesions disrupt the perforant path, resulting in nearly 60% loss of synaptic input to the granule cells of the dentate gyrus. However, beginning as early as a few days after the lesion, new synapses are formed and within two months virtually all the lost inputs are replaced (Matthews *et al.*, 1976). Following fimbria-fornix lesions, synaptic replacement occurs as a result of the growth of fibers from the adrenergic neurons in the superior cervical ganglion into the denervated region (Moore *et al.*, 1977). In the case of entorhinal damage, the new synapses originate from the cholinergic cells of the medial septum, from glutaminergic commissural-associational pyramidal cells and, to a lesser extent, from neurons of the contralateral entorhinal cortex (Lynch *et al.*, 1972; Steward *et al.*, 1990).

In the aged rat, lesion-induced compensatory sprouting in the hippocampus occurs more slowly (Hoff *et al.*, 1982) and, in some cases, less completely (Cotman and Scheff, 1979) than in younger animals. Glucocorticoids suppress hippocampal sprouting in young animals in a dose-related manner (Scheff, Benardo and Cotman, 1980b). In young adult rats maintained on high glucocorticoid levels (mimicking those seen in the aged rats) hippocampal sprouting was significantly reduced following lesions of either the fimbria-fornix (DeKosky *et al.*, 1984) or the entorhinal cortex (Scheff *et al.*, 1980b; Scheff and DeKosky, 1983). Thus, the elevated glucocorticoid levels apparent in the aged rat are associated with reduced synaptogenesis in response to local neuronal damage. These data raise the possibility that in addition to regulating the extent of tissue damage, glucocorticoids may actively dampen the compensatory response of surviving neurons in the presence of neuropathology.

Recently, Poirier *et al.* (1990) used an *in vitro* translation assay to screen total hippocampal RNAs from control and entorhinal cortex lesioned animals. They found that at least seven mRNAs showed altered prevalence 14 days post-lesion. Subsequent analysis showed increased expression of glial fibrillary acidic protein (GFAP) and apolipoprotein E. The increase in GFAP is predictable in light of the glial hypentrophy that accompanies neuronal damage. Of perhaps greater interest is the increase in apolipoprotein E, which facilitates the transport of cholesterol into and out of cells (Mahley, 1988). In response to sciatic nerve damage, macrophages synthesize and secrete large amounts of apolipoprotein E in order to scavenge cholesterol from neuronal debris (Boyles *et al.*, 1985, 1989; Mahley, 1988).

In a time course study, Poirier *et al.* (1991) demonstrated that GFAP mRNA levels peak as early as two days following entorhinal cortex lesions, whereas apolipoprotein E mRNA levels are maximal only six days post-lesion. The increase in GFAP induction corresponds to the early phase of neuronal degeneration and synaptic loss, whereas apolipoprotein E induction is maximal during the acute phase of reactive synaptogenesis (Scheff *et al.*, 1980a; Hoff *et al.*, 1982; Steward and Vinsant, 1983). Again, these findings support the idea that apolipoprotein E is involved in the formation of replacement synapses.

Scheff and DeKosky (1983) suggested that the reduced sprouting in the presence of elevated glucocorticoid levels might occur because of the anti-inflammatory effects of the glucocorticoids (see Munck *et al.*, 1984). Recent findings have suggested a possible mechanism by which circulating glucocorticoids might modulate the synaptogenic response. The apolipoprotein E complex exerts its effects by binding with a low density lipoprotein receptor located on neurons. It is through the binding with the LDL receptor that apolipoprotein E is able to transport scavenged cholesterol into the surviving neurons. Poirier and his colleagues have recently found that hippocampal LDL receptor mRNA is increased following lesions to the entorhinal cortex and that this effect is blocked by corticosterone administration. These findings provide direct evidence for a mechanism whereby glucocorticoids could interfere with compensatory responses of surviving neurons following neuronal damage.

The HPA axis and brain aging: summary

The influence of adrenal steroids on hippocampus in later life illustrates the manner in which peripheral endocrine signals can modulate the process of brain aging. In the case of the adrenal glucocorticoids, there appear to be at least three distinct ways in which these steroids modulate hippocampal function in the aged rat. In each case, we assume that the effects are associated with a loss of function.[1,2]

1. Glucocorticoids can regulate the process of neuron loss.
2. Glucocorticoids alter electrophysiological signal conduction within hippocampal neurons.
3. Glucocorticoids can dampen compensatory responses (e.g., reactive synaptogenesis) of surviving hippocampal neurons to neuron loss.

Individual differences in HPA activity and brain aging

Endocrine and psychological responses to stress are notoriously variable across individuals of the same species. This variation often emerges as an important predictor of vulnerability to stress-induced pathology. Over the course of the past years we have been attempting to understand the neurobiological mechanisms underlying individual differences in HPA responses to stress. In these studies we have used the infant handling paradigm developed some time ago by a number of developmental psychobiologists (e.g., Ader and Grota, 1969; Levine, 1957, 1962, 1970; Levine *et al.*, 1967). In these experiments rat pups are taken from their nest and handled daily for 15 min over the first three weeks of life. The animals are weaned on day 22 of life and handled (H) and nonhandled (NH) rats are then housed under similar conditions until maturity.

As adults, handled (H) animals secrete less corticosterone and show a faster return to basal corticosterone levels following the termination of stress than do nonhandled (NH) animals (Hess *et al.*, 1969; Levine, 1957, 1962; Levine *et al.*, 1967; Meaney *et al.*, 1985a, 1988b, 1989, 1991a, 1991b). These differences are apparent as late as 24-26 months of age (Meaney *et al.*, 1988b, 1991), indicating that the handling effect persists over the entire life of the animal. The differences in HPA function are

---

[1] In addition to these effects, glucocorticoids also regulate neurotransmission in a number of brain regions through their effects on transmitter turnover, receptor biosynthesis, and post-receptor effector systems (see McEwen *et al.*, 1986; Meyer, 1986 for reviews). It is very likely that altered hippocampal function associated with elevated glucocorticoid levels in the aged animal is associated with an effect on neurotransmitter function.

[2] Glucocorticoids (as the name implies) are potent regulators of carbohydrate metabolism (Baxter and Tyrrell, 1987). Hypercorticoid states are associated with an altered ability to metabolize glucose, decreased sensitivity to insulin, ketosis, and lyposis, resulting in increased fat levels. Fat involution in the liver is markedly increased in hypercorticoid states and is striking in old rats with elevated glucocorticoid levels (Viau and Meaney, unpublished observation). Quite apart from the direct effects on brain cells, it is also worth considering the effects of these changes in peripheral metabolism on brain function.

not due to changes in adrenal sensitivity to ACTH (Grota 1975; Meaney *et al.*, 1989b) or in pituitary sensitivity to CRH (Meaney *et al.*, 1989b). Moreover, there are no differences between H and NH animals in the metabolic clearance rate for corticosterone (Grota 1975; Meaney *et al.*, 1989b). Rather, the difference lies in the fact that the NH animals show increased secretion of corticosterone both during and following stress.

Young adult H and NH animals do not differ in levels of CBG, the principal plasma binder for corticosterone (Meaney *et al.*, 1985a, 1991b) or in free corticosterone levels (Meaney *et al.*, 1991b). This finding is of considerable importance since brain uptake of corticosterone appears to approximate the non-CBG bound (free + albumin-bound) portion of the steroid (Partridge *et al.*, 1983). Thus, differences in total corticosterone are likely predictive of differences in brain uptake of the steroid. One further point of importance concerns the specificity of this difference. Young adult H and NH animals do not differ in basal corticosterone levels at any time point over the diurnal cycle (Meaney *et al.*, 1988b, 1989, 1991b). Thus, the difference between the two groups of animals is specific to conditions of stress and is not seen under normal, resting conditions. This finding also indicates that differences in HPA activity observed during stress cannot be accounted for by differences in pre-stress, basal glucocorticoid levels.

H and NH animals also differ in plasma ACTH and ACTH secretagogue responses to stress. Levels of CRH-like bioactivity (Zarrow *et al.*, 1972) and plasma ACTH (Meaney *et al.*, 1989b) are higher both during and following stress in NH animals. These findings suggest that the mechanism(s) for differences between H and NH animals is located above the level of the pituitary and that the post-stress difference, at least, may be related to differential sensitivity of CNS negative feedback processes.

On the basis of the relative hypersecretion of ACTH and corticosterone by NH animals, we wondered whether H and NH animals might differ in negative-feedback sensitivity to circulating glucocorticoids. We (Meaney *et al.*, 1989b) tested this idea using a classical negative-feedback paradigm based on the finding that high levels of circulating glucorticoids feed back onto the brain and/or pituitary to inhibit subsequent HPA activity (see Keller-Wood and Dallman, 1984). Such delayed, negative feedback persists for hours following exposure to elevated glucocorticoid levels. In these experiments, H and NH animals were injected with one of five doses of either corticosterone or dexamethasone 3 hours prior to a 20-min immobilization stress. Both glucocorticoids were more effective in suppressing stress-induced HPA responses in the H animals (i.e., the ID_{50} for both corticosterone and dexamethasone was 5-10 times lower in the H animals). These data suggest that indeed the H animals are more sensitive to the negative-feedback effects of circulating glucocorticoids on HPA activity.

Since this delayed form of negative feedback is likely mediated by the binding of corticosterone to soluble intracellular receptors, we have measured both mineralocorticoid and glucocorticoid receptor sites in selected brain regions and pituitary of young adult H and NH animals (Meaney and Aitken, 1985; Meaney *et al.*, 1985a, 1985b, 1987, 1988b, 1989b, 1991a, 1991b; Sarrieau *et al.*, 1988a). The results of these studies have demonstrated that there are significant and regionally-specific differences in glucocorticoid receptor binding capacity as a function of handling. H animals show increased glucocorticoid receptor binding capacity in the hippocampus, but not in septum, amygdala, hypothalamus, or pituitary. The difference in the receptor binding data is clearly related to the number of receptor sites, and not to the affinity of the receptor for ^{3}H- radioligand, RU 28362. Moreover, the difference occurs in glucocorticoid receptors, but not the mineralocorticoid receptor sites (measured using either radiolabeled aldosterone or corticosterone + 50-fold excess of cold RU 28362).

We (Meaney *et al.*, 1989b) have demonstrated that this difference in hippocampal glucocorticoid receptor density is related to the more efficient suppression of post-stress HPA activity in the H animals. Chronic administration of corticosterone results in a 30-45% down-regulation of hippocampal glucocorticoid receptor binding sites (Sapolsky *et al.*, 1984b; Tornello *et al.*, 1982). The effect is highly specific to the hippocampus, such that receptor binding capacity in the hypothalamus and pituitary are unaffected. In this experiment we treated H animals for 5 days with corticosterone, and allowed 2 days for steroid clearance. Hippocampal glucocorticoid receptor density was down-regulated in the H + corticosterone animals to levels that were indistinguishable from those of NH animals, and significantly less than that of the H + vehicle animals. There were no differences in glucocorticoid receptor density in the hypothalamus or pituitary. When the animals in these groups were exposed to a 20-min immobilization stress, we found that the H + corticosterone animals, like the NH animals, hypersecreted corticosterone 60 and 120 min post-stress in comparison to the H + vehicle control animals. These data suggest that the difference in negative-feedback efficiency between H and NH is related to the differences in hippocampal glucocorticoid receptor density. Thus, the chronic corticosterone treatment reversed both the handling-induced increase in hippocampal glucocorticoid receptor binding capacity and the difference in post-stress HPA activity. It appears, then, that the increase in glucocorticoid receptor sites in the hippocampus is a critical feature for the handling effect on HPA function. The increase in receptor density appears to increase the sensitivity of the hippocampus to circulating glucocorticoids, enhancing the efficacy of negative-feedback inhibition over HPA activity, and serving to reduce post-stress secretion of ACTH and corticosterone in H animals.

Aging rats lose hippocampal corticosteroid receptors, become insensitive to glucocorticoid negative-feedback regulation (Sapolsky *et al.*, 1986b), and hypersecrete corticosterone under both basal and post-stress conditions. Throughout life, however, H animals have significantly higher hippocampal glucocorticoid receptors than do NH animals (Meaney *et al.*, 1988b, 1991a, 1992b), although both groups do show a loss of receptors. As expected on the basis of these receptor data, we found that the age-related HPA deficits were far less pronounced in the H rats (Meaney *et al.*, 1988b, 1991). At each age tested, the H animals secreted less corticosterone during restraint stress and terminated corticosterone secretion following stress sooner than did the NH rats.

Moreover, the age-related rise in basal corticosterone levels, often seen in aged rats, was observed in the NH, but not the H animals (Meaney *et al.*, 1988b, 1991a, 1991b). There was about a two-fold increase in basal corticosterone levels in the aged NH animals in the PM phase of the light cycle and about a 40% increase during the AM phase (Meaney *et al.*, 1991b). However, the difference in the PM phase was amplified by the fact that during this time plasma CBG levels in the aged NH animals were significantly lower than in old H animals or young. The decrease in CBG in the old NH animals was associated with a dramatic elevation in free corticosterone to levels (≈ 3-4 μg/dl) that approximated those achieved during stress. Old H animals showed no such decrease in plasma CBG levels and little or no change in basal corticosterone levels. Again, it should be emphasized that these differences in basal corticosterone and CBG between H and NH animals emerge as a function of age. There are no such differences between 6-month-old H and NH animals.

These findings suggested that over a lifespan, cumulative exposure to the highly catabolic glucocorticoids was greater in the NH animals. We then examined an important neuropathological consequence of this difference. The hippocampus loses neurons with age, particularly in the CA_1 and CA_3 cellfields (see Coleman and Flood, 1987). The hippocampus has extremely high concentrations of corticosteroid receptors and therefore marked sensitivity to glucocorticoids. Thus, the reduced cumulative exposure to glucocorticoids in the H rats suggested that hippocampal degeneration would be less pronounced in these animals and this is exactly what we observed. Among NH animals, but not H animals, there occurred a significant (≈ 40%) loss of neurons with age in both the CA_1 and CA_3 hippocampal cellfields (Meaney *et al.*, 1988b, 1991a). Importantly, H and NH rats did not differ in neuron density at 6 months of age. Rather, handling attenuated the loss of hippocampal neurons occurring at later ages.

The difference in hippocampal cell number between the H and NH animals at the later ages was of functional significance. The hippocampus is known to be of considerable importance in learning and memory, and hippocampal injury profoundly disrupts cognition. These findings suggested that the older H rats, with attenuated cell loss in the hippocampus, should show less evidence of age-related cognitive impairments than older NH rats. Behavioral testing was performed using the Morris swim maze (Morris, 1985), a test of spatial memory in which animals are placed into a large (1.6 m) circular pool of opaque water and must use distal, spatial cues in order to locate a submerged platform onto which they can climb out of the water (rats are proficient, but reluctant swimmers). Spatial memory deficits emerged with age in the NH rats such that the 24-month-old NH animals took significantly longer to locate the platform (i.e., 3-4 times longer) than the 6-month-old animals on all but the first 3 of 18 trials (Meaney *et al.*, 1988b, 1991a). In contrast, among the H rats there were no statistically reliable age differences. The 24-month-old H rats performed as well as the 6-month-old animals. There were no differences in the performance of the H and NH animals at 6 months of age.

In order to control for possible differences in swimming speeds, we also analyzed the data over the last eight trials by scoring the swimming distance before locating the submerged platform. Again, aged NH rats showed a clear, age-related deficit, whereas the H rats did not. Importantly, in subsequent testing, H and NH rats of all ages performed similarly when the platform was made visible by raising it above the water level, indicating that the H/NH differences were due to spatial rather than motor skills. These spatial memory deficits in the older NH animals are probably related to the hippocampal damage seen in these animals, as similar deficits are observed after damage to the dorsal hippocampus (e.g., Morris *et al.*, 1982).

The results of a recent study with hippocampal grafts in aged H and NH animals (Weiner and Meaney, unpublished) are consistent with the idea that compensatory responses to neuronal damage may also vary as a function of differences in hormonal milieu. In this study, we unilaterally lesioned the dorsal hippocampus in 16-18-month-old animals and one week later grafted septal tissue from fetal donors. The growth and survival of the grafts in the old NH rats was markedly reduced compared to the aged H animals. The growth and survival of hippocampal grafts has been shown to be dependent upon the presence of nerve growth factor in the host tissue (Gage and Bjorklund, 1986; Tuszynski *et al.*, 1990). The synthetic glucocorticoid, dexamethasone, suppresses nerve growth factor-induced outgrowth of sympathetic fibers in tissue culture (Unsicker *et al.*, 1978). Glucocorticoids also decrease the synthesis of nerve growth factor mRNA. These findings suggest that glucocorticoids might compromise either neuron survival or regeneration in the presence of an insult by decreasing the synthesis of required growth factors.

Both the present and previous studies have revealed neuroendocrine dysfunction in the aged rat that include glucocorticoid hypersecretion and negative-feedback insensitivity, as well as the loss of hippocampal neurons and glucocorticoid receptors. These deficits form a complex and self-perpetuating cascade (see Sapolsky *et al.*, 1986a); a consequence of glucocorticoid hypersecretion is accelerated neuron loss in the aging hippocampus (including corticosterone-concentrating neurons), and a consequence of hippocampal damage is adrenocortical negative-feedback insensitivity and glucocorticoid hypersecretion. The interaction of these abnormalities occurs with aging in the rat, and is accelerated by conditions which further elevate glucocorticoid levels, such as stress. Neonatal handling reduces the HPA response to stress. Our data show that this effect persists over the lifespan. Moreover, one of the critical features of this effect, that of reducing glucocorticoid concentrations under a variety of conditions, appears to prevent, or at least delay, the degenerative "glucocorticoid cascade" that characterizes aging in the rat (see Sapolsky *et al.*, 1986a).

The diminished rate of hippocampal neuron loss in the aging H rats probably reflects the lower cumulative lifetime exposure to glucocorticoids. It should be noted that this outcome is the product of two apparently opposing trends. While the increased concentrations of hippocampal glucocorticoid receptors are related to the enhanced negative-feedback sensitivity and decreased glucocorticoid secretion in the H rats, the same high receptor concentrations could conceivably sensitize the hippocampus to the endangering effects of glucocorticoids. In this instance, the decreased secretion apparently outweighs the risk of increased target sensitivity, perhaps by ensuring that the prolonged glucocorticoid exposure necessary for the endangering effects does not occur. It should be noted that under normal resting conditions only about 10-15% of the hippocampal glucocorticoid receptor population is occupied by hormone (Meaney *et al.*, 1988a; Reul and DeKloet, 1985; Reul *et al*,. 1987). Thus, as glucocorticoid levels rise with age it is the change in hormone levels rather than receptor density that determines the increase in the corticoid signal.

Thus, an environmental manipulation occurring early in life results in a sequence of changes that endures throughout the lifespan, with dramatic attenuation of some of the deficits typical of aging. These findings cast considerable light upon the regulatory relationships linking adrenocortical secretory patterns, hippocampal glucocorticoid receptor concentrations, and hippocampal pathology and dysfunction. In addition, they demonstrate that relatively subtle individual differences in early experience can alter profoundly the quality of aging years later. This underscores the importance of developmental critical periods and explains a possible source of variability of aging studies. It is important that H and NH animals do not differ in hippocampal neuron number and spatial memory ability at 6 months of age. Rather, the difference emerges over time as the function of an interaction with age. Thus, the H/NH difference in these measures at later ages represents a true retardation of the aging process in the H rats.

These findings, taken together with the earlier studies of Landfield, suggest that in a normal population of laboratory rats, individual differences in HPA activity should serve as a predictor of age-related hippocampal pathology. We (Issa *et al.*, 1990) further examined this question by screening a large sample of aged (22-28 months) rats using a test of spatial memory. If HPA dysfunction is associated with hippocampal pathology and not merely with advanced age, then we would expect that a sample of aged, cognitively-impaired (ACI) and aged, cognitively-unimpaired (ACU) should differ considerably in HPA activity. We used the Morris water maze (a test of spatial memory) to screen over 100 aged animals, in order to select aged animals that were either cognitively impaired or unimpaired (> 2 SD or < 0.5 SD from the mean of 6-month-old animals, respectively). According to this criterion, about 30% of the animals were designated as ACI and a comparable percentage as ACU (underscoring the extreme variation in cognitive decline in aged rats). These data are comparable to previous studies using this screening procedure (Gage *et al.*, 1984; Pelleymounter *et al.*, 1990). Interestingly, both groups of aged animals showed some loss of hippocampal neurons; however, the decrease in neuron density was substantially greater in the ACI rats.

The ACI animals showed increased plasma ACTH and corticosterone levels under both basal and post-stress conditions, whereas HPA activity in the aged-unimpaired animals did not differ from 6-month-old controls. Interestingly, while both aged groups showed a loss of hippocampal glucocorticoid receptors (with no change in hypothalamic or pituitary receptor density), the loss was significantly greater in the ACI animals. The ACI rats also showed a significant decrease in hippocampal mineralocorticoid receptor density. These findings demonstrate the overall loss of hippocampal corticosteroid receptors in the ACI animals. The pattern of data in this study was comparable to that of the previous handling studies, where the old H animals resembled the ACU rats in the Issa *et al.* study. Taken together with the findings of the Landfield studies, these data strongly suggest that increased glucocorticoid levels are selectively associated with the occurrence of hippocampal pathology and impaired cognition in later life.

Stress and brain aging

Several decades ago, Selye (e.g., Selye, 1950) suggested that increased exposure to stress could accelerate the degeneration that normally accompanies aging. Increased exposure to the highly catabolic glucocorticoids now appears to be a major factor mediating this relationship. However, from the preceding studies it appears that it would be unwise to accept the idea that stress will necessarily alter the course of brain aging without also considering the nature of the individual's endocrine response to threatening stimuli. In both the handling studies as well as those with "normal" populations of laboratory rats we have commonly seen aged animals which do not differ from young adult animals in HPA responses to stress. These animals also show no evidence of hippocampal dysfunction.

From these studies it would seem that stress can accentuate hippocampal damage, but that this relationship is most likely to be apparent in animals where there is evidence of exaggerated HPA activity in response to stress. Thus, the relationship between stress and brain aging is best understood if one factors into the equation some knowledge of individual differences in endocrine responses to stress. Moreover, we must also consider the magnitude of the increase in basal HPA activity. Under resting conditions, aged NH rats show free corticosterone levels that are comparable to those occurring in response to stress ($\approx$ 3-4 μg/dl). In these animals glucocorticoid-related hippocampal dysfunction need not be related to the presence of stressful stimuli; the elevation in the basal levels is very likely sufficient to account for hippocampal damage.[3]

---

[3] Of course this argument may largely be a case of semantics. It is possible that the elevated "basal" levels of corticosterone observed in aged rats occurs in response to a metabolic disturbance (e.g., altered carbohydrate metabolism), that could clearly be considered as a stressor. Ultimately, these issues have less to do with what one considers to be a stressor than with clearly defining the physiological conditions that lead to increased HPA activity.

HPA function in human brain aging

In general, increased HPA activity is not associated with aging in humans. However, as in the rat, elevated glucocorticoid levels do seem to accompany age-related neuropathology. In studies with multiple samples (as is required in studies of hormones that show circadian rhythms), cortisol levels were found to be significantly higher in SDAT patients compared with controls. Davis *et al.* (1986) previously reported significantly higher cortisol levels in SDAT patients, an effect that was most consistent during the late PM–early AM phase of the cycle (i.e., 0200 h to 0900 h). These authors also reported the 0900 h sample discriminated best between SDAT patients and healthy controls. In our own study, we (Nair *et al.*, submitted) found that differences in cortisol levels were more or less consistent across the 24-hour cycle and that this was true for both males and females. Moreover, the magnitude of the difference in basal cortisol levels between SDAT patients and controls was substantial (30 to 52% for males and 57 to 102% for females). These reports also indicated that the pattern of cortisol levels over the 24-hour cycle was very similar in SDAT patients and healthy controls. These findings are consistent with previous reports that despite changes in secretory patterns and some evidence of phase shifts, a circadian rhythm in hormone levels is preserved in later life. These findings suggest that while CNS factors involved in the drive over hypothalamic-pituitary-adrenal activity may be altered in Alzheimer's disease, the signals from the circadian pacemakers which govern the pattern of hormone levels is unchanged.

Interestingly, there may also be changes in plasma CBG levels in SDAT patients. In preliminary, studies we (Meaney *et al.*, 1989c) found a significant (–50%) decrease in plasma CBG levels and increased (≈ 200%) free cortisol concentrations in SDAT patients. Thus, measures of total cortisol levels may actually have underestimated the magnitude of the elevated glucocorticoid signal in SDAT patents.

The cause of the increase in basal cortisol levels in SDAT patients is not clear. Resistance to dexamethasone suppression has been reported in a significant number of dementia patients (reviewed in Sapolsky, 1987), which might indicate a dampening of glucocorticoid negative-feedback control over HPA function. The recent report of increased CRF-like immunoreactivity in the paraventricular nucleus of the hypothalamus (PVN) is consistent with this view (Powers *et al.*, 1987), since this region contains the cell bodies of CRF neurons that project into the hypophysial portal system of the anterior pituitary. Bissette *et al.* (1985) found small and non-significant elevation in CRF-like immunoreactivity between Alzheimer's patients and controls. However, this analysis was performed using the whole hypothalamus.

Within the hypothalamus it is only a subpopulation of the CRF-immunoreactive neurons, localized in the medial-parvocellular region, that project to the median eminence and thereby regulate ACTH release (see Anton, 1986; Swanson *et al.*, 1987 for reviews). Moreover, this population of CRF-immunoreactive neurons are unique in their sensitivity to glucocorticoids (Swanson *et al.*, 1987). For the study of possible feedback deficits, this is the most relevant population of neurons and it is not hard to imagine that analysis of whole hypothalamus might have masked differences occurring with this region, such as those detected by Powers *et al.* (1987).

These findings have led to the hypothesis that increased glucocorticoid levels might promote the loss of hippocampal neurons in later life in humans (see Sapolsky, 1986a). It is interesting that hippocampal neuron loss is a hallmark of Alzheimer's disease. Several years ago Sapolsky and Meaney (1986) made a concerted effort to examine the glucocorticoid receptor binding in post-mortem human brain tissue. We (Sarrieau *et al.*, 1988b) have identified the receptor in biopsy samples of human temporal cortex, but unfortunately it appears as though the glucocorticoid receptor decays quickly following death in the primate brain. This question will likely need to be assessed with measures of changes in receptor mRNAs (e.g., Peiffer *et al.*, in press), and these studies are currently in progress. To date, the meager evidence on the HPA axis and neuropathology in humans is, at best, consistent with the data from the rodent studies. It is certainly worth mentioning, however, that the evidence to date also suggests that prolonged exposure to elevated glucocorticoid levels can damage the primate hippocampus (see Sapolsky *et al.*, 1990). The results of the early experience studies would seem to provide yet one more reason for a more humane and intelligent approach to the needs of our children.

Finally, it is certainly not our intention to argue that the glucocorticoids are the sole, or even necessarily the principal regulator of hippocampal pathology in the aged mammal. Rather, the purpose of this review was to illustrate the manner in which peripheral endocrine signals might act as modulators of brain aging. Certainly one challenge for the current study of brain aging is to identify any potential endocrine signals, perhaps certain growth factors, that might promote neuron survival and preserve cognitive function.

References

Ader, R. and Grota, L. J. (1969). Effects of early experience on adrenocortical reactivity. *Physiol. Behav.* **4**: 303-305.

Aitken, D. H. and Meaney, M. J. (1991). Temporally graded, age-related impairments in spatial memory in the rat. *Neurobiol. Aging*.

Anton, F. A. (1986). Hypothalamic control of ACTH secretion: advances since the discovery of 41-residue corticotropin-releasing factor. *Endo. Rev.* **7**: 351-370.

Balldin, J., Gottfries, C. G., Karlsson, I., *et al.* (1983). Dexamethasone suppression test and serum prolactin in dementia disorders. *Brit. J. Psychiat.* **143**: 277-281.

Bartus, R. T. and Dean, R. L. (1987). Behavioral models of aging in nonhuman primates. In: *Animal Models of Dementia*, ed., J. T. Coyle, Liss, New York, pp. 69-95.

Baxter, J. D. and Tyrrell, J. B. (1987). The adrenal cortex. In: *Endocrinology and Metabolism*, eds., P. Felig, J. D. Baxter, A. E. Broadus and L. A. Frohman, McGraw-Hill, New York, pp. 385-511.

Beaumont, K. and Fanestil, D. D. (1983). Characterization of rat brain aldosterone receptors reveals high affinity for corticosterone. *Endocrinology* **113**: 2043-2051.

Benston, J., Rena, M. R., Winter, J. and Wilson, G. (1978). Steroids and apparent cerebral atrophy on computed tomography scans. *J. Comp. Ass. Tomography* **2**: 16-23.

Bissette, G., Reynolds, G. P., Kjlts, C. D. and Nemeroff, C. (1985). Corticotropin-releasing factor-like immunoreactivity in senile dementia of the Alzheimer type. *JAMA* **254**: 3067-3069.

Boyles, J. K., Pitas, R. E., Wilson, E., Mahley, R. W. and Taylor J. M. (1985). Apolipoprotein E associated with astrocytic glia of the central nervous system and with non-myelinating glia of the peripheral nervous system. *J. Clin. Invest.* **76**: 1501-1513.

Boyles, J. K., Zoellner, C. D., Anderson, L. J., Kosick, L. M., Pitas, R. E., Weisgraber, K. H., Hui, D. Y., Mahley, R. W., Gebiecke-Haeter, P. J., Ignatius, M. J. and Shooter, E. M. (1989). A role for apolipoprotein E, apolipoprotein A-1, and low density lipoprotein receptors in cholesterol transport during regeneration and remyelination of rat sciatic nerve. *J. Clin. Invest.* **83**: 1015-1031.

Bradbury, M. and Dallman, M. F. (1989). Effects of type 1 and type 2 glucocorticoid receptor antagonists on ACTH levels in the PM. *Soc. Neurosci. Abst.* **19**: 716.

Brett, L. P., Chong, G. S., Coyle, S. and Levine, S. (1983). The pituitary-adrenal response to novel stimulation and ether stress in young adult and aged rats. *Neurobiol. Aging* **4**: 133-138.

Coirini, H., Magarinos, A. M., DeNicola, A. F., Rainbow, T. C. and McEwen, B. S. (1985). Further studies of brain aldosterone binding sites employing new mineralocorticoid and glucocorticoid receptor markers *in vitro*. *Brain Res.* **361**: 212-217.

Coleman, P. D. and Flood, D. G. (1987). Neuron numbers and dendritic extent in normal aging and Alzheimer's disease. *Neurobiol. Aging* **8**: 521-545.

Cotman, C. W. and Scheff, S. W. (1979). Compensatory synapse growth in aged animals after neuronal death. *Mech. Aging Dev.* **9**: 103-117.

Dallman, M. F., Akana, S., Cascio, C. S., Darlington, D. N., Jacobson, L. and Levin, N. (1987). Regulation of ACTH secretion: Variations on a theme of B. *Rec. Prog. Horm. Res.* **43**: 113-173.

Davis, K. L., Davis, B. M. and Greenwald, B. S. (1986). Cortisol and Alzheimer's disease, I: Basal studies. *Am. J. Psychiatry* **143**: 300-305.

DeKosky, S. T., Scheff, S. W. and Cotman, C. W. (1984). Elevated corticosterone levels: A possible cause of reduced axon sprouting in aged animals. *Neuroendocrinology* **38**: 33-38.

Dilman, V. (1981). *The Law of Deviation of Homeostasis and Diseases of Aging*. Boston, John Wiley.

Emadian, S. M., Luttge, W. G. and Densmore, C. L. (1986). Chemical differentiation of Type I and Type II receptors for adrenal steroids in brain cytosol. *J. Steroid Biochem*. 24: 953-961.

Feldman, S. and Conforti, N. (1976). Feedback effects of dexamethasone on adrenocortical responses in rats with fornix lesions. *Horm. Res*. **7**: 56-60.

Feldman, S. and Conforti, N. (1980). Participation of the dorsal hippocampus in the glucocorticoid negative-feedback effect on adrenocortical activity. *Neuroendocrinology* **30**: 52-55.

Fischette, C. T., Komisurak, B. R., Ediner, H. M., Feder, H. H. and Siegal, A. (1980). Differential fornix ablations and the circadian rhythmicity of adrenal corticosterone secretion. *Brain Res*. **195**: 373-380.

Funder, J. W. and Sheppard, K. (1987). Adrenocortical steroids and the brain. *Ann. Rev. Physiol*. **49**: 397-412.

Gage, F. H. and Bjorklund, A. (1986). Enhanced graft survival in the hippocampus following selective denervation. *Neurosci*. **17**: 89-98.

Gage, F. H., Kelly, P. A. T. and Bjorklund, A. (1984). Regional changes in brain glucose metabolism reflect cognitive impairments in aged rats. *J. Neurosci*. **4**: 2856-2865.

Gala, R. R. and Westphal, U. (1965). Corticosteroid-binding globulin in the rat: studies on the sex differences. *Endocrinology* **77**: 841-851.

Gibbs, D. M. (1986). Vasopressin and oxytocin: hypothalamic modulators of the stress response. *Psychoneuroendocrinology* **11**: 131-140.

Grota, L. J. (1975). Effects of early experience on the metabolism and production of corticosterone in rats. *Dev. Psychobiol*. **9**: 211-215.

Heinz, E. R., Martinez, J. and Haenggeli, A. (1977). Reversibility of cerebral atrophy in anorexia nervosa and Cushing's syndrome. *J. Comp. Ass. Tomography* **1**: 415-418.

Herman, J. P., Schafer, M. K.-H., Young, E. A., Thompson, R., Douglass, J., Akil, H. and Watson, S. J. (1989). Evidence for hippocampal regulation of neuroendocrine neurons of the hypothalamo-pituitary-adrenocortical axis. *J. Neurosci*. **9**: 3072-3082.

Hess, G. D. and Reigle, G. D. (1970). Adrenocortical responsiveness to stress and ACTH in aging rats. *J. Gerontol*. **25**: 253-270.

Hess, J. L., Denenberg, V. H., Zarrow, M. X. and Pfeifer, W. D. (1969). Modification of the corticosterone response curve as a function of handling in infancy. *Physiol. Behav*. **4**: 109-112.

Hoff, S. F., Scheff, S. W., Benardo, L. S. and Cotman, C. W. (1982). Lesions-induced synaptogenesis in the dentate gyrus of aged rats: I. Loss of reacquisition of normal synaptic density. *J. Comp. Neurol*. **205**: 246-252.

Homer, H. and Sapolsky, R. M. (1988). Glucocorticoids decrease glucose transport in cultured hippocampal neurons. *Soc. Neurosci. Abst*. **11**: 372.

Issa, A., Gauthier, S. and Meaney, M. J. (1990). Hypothalamic-pituitary-adrenal activity in aged cognitively impaired and cognitively unimpaired aged rats. *J. Neurosci.* **10**: 3247-3254.

Joels, M. and De Kloet, E. R. (1989). Effect of glucocorticoids and norepinephrine on excitability in the hippocampus. *Science* **245**: 1502-1504.

Jones, M. T., Gillham, B., Greenstein, B. D., Beckford, U. and Holmes, M. C. (1982). Feedback actions of adrenal steroid hormones. In: *Current Topics in Neuroendocrinology, Vol. 2,* eds., D. Ganten and D. Pfaff, Springer, New York, pp. 45-68.

Keller-Wood, M. and Dallman, M. (1984). Corticosteroid inhibition of ACTH secretion. *Endo. Rev.* **5**: 1-24.

Kerr, D. S., Campbell, L. W., Hao, S.-Y. and Landfield, P. W. (1989). Corticosteroid modulation of hippocampal potentials: increased effect with aging. *Science* **245**: 1505-1509.

Krozowski, Z. S. and Funder, J. W. (1983). Renal mineralocorticoid receptors and hippocampal corticosterone binding species have intrinsic steroid specificity. *Proc. Nat. Acad. Sci. U.S.A.* **80**: 6056-6060.

Landfield, P., Waymire, J. and Lynch, G. (1978). Hippocampal aging and adrenocorticoids: a quantitative correlation. *Science* **202**: 1098-1101.

Landfield, P., Baskin, R. K. and Pitler, T. A. (1981). Brain-aging correlates: retardation by hormonal-pharmacological treatments. *Science* **214**: 581-583.

Lee, K. D., Stanford, E. J., Cotman, C. W. and Lynch, G. S. (1977). Ultrastructural evidence for boutin proliferation in partially deafferented dentate gyrus in the adult rat. *Exp. Brain Res.* **29**: 475-485.

Levine, S. (1970). The pituitary-adrenal system and the developing brain. *Prog. Brain Res.* **32**: 79-102.

Levine, S. (1957). Infantile experience and resistance to physiological stress. *Science* **126**: 405-406.

Levine, S. (1962). Plasma-free corticosteroid response to electric shock in rats stimulated in infancy. *Science* **135**: 795-796.

Levine, S., Haltmeyer, G. C., Karas, G. G. and Denenberg, V. H. (1967). Physiological and behavioral effects of infantile stimulation. *Physiol. Behav.* **2**: 55-63.

Linton, E. A., Tilders, F. J. H., Hodgkinson, S., Berkenbosch, F., Vermes, I. and Lowry, P. J. (1985). Stress-induced secretion of adrenocorticotropin in rats is inhibited by antisera to corticotropin-releasing factor and vasopressin. *Endocrinology* **116**: 966-970.

Lynch, G., Matthews, D. A., Mosko, S., Parks, T. and Cotman, C. W. (1972). Induced acetylcholinesterase rich layer in rat dentate gyrus following entorhinal lesions. *Brain Res.* **42**: 311-323.

Mahley, R. W. (1988). Apolipoprotein E: cholesterol transport protein with expanding role in cell biology. *Science* **240**: 622-630.

Matthews, D. A., Cotman, C. W. and Lynch, G. (1976). An electron microscopic study of lesion-induced synaptogenesis in the dentate gyrus of the adult rat. *Brain Res.* **115**: 1-41.

McEwen, B. S. (1982). Glucocorticoids and hippocampus: receptors in search of a function. In: *Current Topics in Neuroendocrinology, Vol. 2,* eds., D. Ganten and D. Pfaff, Springer, New York, pp. 1-22.

McEwen, B. S., DeKloet, E. R. and Rostene, W. H. (1986). Adrenal steroid receptors and actions in the nervous system. *Physiol. Rev.* **66**: 1121-1150.

Meaney, M. J. and Aitken, D. H. (1985). The effects of early postnatal handling on the development of hippocampal glucocorticoid receptors: temporal parameters. *Dev. Brain Res.* **22**: 301-304.

Meaney, M. J., Aitken, D. H., Bodnoff, S. R., Iny, L. J. and Sapolsky, R. M. (1985a). The effects of postnatal handling on the development of the glucocorticoid receptor systems and stress recovery in the rat. *Prog. Neuropsychopharm. Biol. Psychiat.* **7**: 731-734.

Meaney, M. J., Aitken, D. H., Bodnoff, S. R., Iny, L. J., Tatarewicz, J. E. and Sapolsky, R. M. (1985b). Early, postnatal handling alters glucocorticoid receptor concentrations in selected brain regions. *Behav. Neurosci.* **99**: 760-765.

Meaney, M. J., Aitken, D. H. and Sapolsky, R. M. (1987). Thyroid hormones influence the development of hippocampal glucocorticoid receptors in the rat: a mechanism for the effects of postnatal handling on the development of the adrenocortical stress response. *Neuroendocrinology* **45**: 278-283.

Meaney, M. J., Viau, V., Bhatnagar, S. and Aitken, D. H. (1988a). Occupancy and translocation of hippocampal glucocorticoid receptors during and following stress. *Brain Res.* **445**: 198-203.

Meaney, M. J., Aitken, D. H., Bhatnagar, S., Van Berkel, C. and Sapolsky, R. M. (1988b). Postnatal handling attenuates neuroendocrine, anatomical, and cognitive impairments related to the aged hippocampus. *Science* **238**: 766-768.

Meaney, M. J., Viau, V., Aitken, D. H. and Bhatnagar, S. (1989a). Glucocorticoid receptors in brain and pituitary of the lactating rat. *Physiol. Behav.* **43**: 209-212.

Meaney, M. J., Aitken, D. H., Sharma, S., Viau, V. and Sarrieau, A. (1989b). Postnatal handling increases hippocampal type II glucocorticoid receptors and enhances adrenocortical negative-feedback efficacy in the rat. *Neuroendocrinology* **50**: 597-604.

Meaney, M. J., Sharma, M., Sharma, S., Thakur, M., Quirion, R., Sapolsky, R. M. and Nair, N. P. V. (1989c). Hypothalamic-pituitary-adrenal function in Alzheimer patients and aged controls. *Soc. Neurosci. Abstr.* **15**: 1043.

Meaney, M. J., Aitken, D. H. and Sapolsky, R. M. (1991a). Environmental regulation of the adrenocortical stress response in female rats and its implications for individual differences in aging. *Neurobiol. Aging*.

Meaney, M. J., Aitken, D. H., Sharma, S. and Viau, V. (1991b). Basal ACTH, corticosterone, and corticosterone-binding globulin levels over the diurnal cycle, and hippocampal type I and type II corticosteroid receptors in young and old, handled and nonhandled rats. *Neuroendocrinology*.

Meyer, J. S. (1986). Biochemical effects of corticosteroids on neural tissues. *Physiol. Rev.* **65**: 970-1019.

Moore, R. Y., Bjorklund, A. and Stenevi, U. (1977). Plastic changes in the adrenergic innervation of the rat septal area in response to denervation. *Brain Res.* **33**: 13-35.

Morris, R. G. M. (1985). An attempt to dissociate "spatial mapping" and "working memory" theories of hippocampal functioning. In: *Neurobiology of the Hippocampus*, ed., W. Seifert, Academic Press, New York, pp. 405-432.

Morris, R. G. M., Garrard, P., Rawlins, J. N. P. and O'Keefe, J. (1982). Place navigation impaired in rats with hippocampal lesions. *Nature* **297**: 681-683.

Munck, A., Guyre, P. M. and Holbrook, N. J. (1984). Physiological functions of glucocorticoids in stress and their relations to pharmacological actions. *Endo. Rev.* **5**: 25-44.

Nair, N. P. V., Sharma, M., Thakur, M., Schwartz, G., Ghadirian, A., Quirion, R. and Meaney, M. J. (submitted). Circadian rhythms of cortisol and melatonin in senile dementia of Alzheimer's type (SDAT).

Nakane, T., Aughya, T., Kanie, N. and Hollander, C. S. (1985). Evidence for the role of endogenous corticotropin-releasing factor in cold, ether, immobilization, and a traumatic stress. *Proc. Nat. Acad. Sci. U.S.A.* **82**: 1247-1251.

Okuno, T., Ito, M., Konishi, Y., Yosbioka, Y. and Nakano, Y. (1980). Cerebral atrophy following ACTH therapy. *J. Comp. Ass. Tomography* **4**: 20-23.

Packan, D. and Sapolsky, R. M. (1990). Glucocorticoid endangerment of the hippocampus: tissue, steroid, and receptor specificity. *Neuroendocrinology* **51**: 613-618.

Partridge, W. M., Sakiyama, R. and Judd, H. L. (1983). Protein-bound corticosterone in human serum is selectively transported into rat brain and liver *in vivo*. *J. Clin. Endocrinol. Metabol.* **57**: 160-166.

Peiffer, A., Barden, N. and Meaney, M. J. (1991). Age-related changes in glucocorticoid receptor binding and mRNA levels in the rat brain and pituitary. *Neurobiol. Aging.*

Pelleymounter, M. A., Beatty, G. and Gallagher, M. (1990). Hippocampal ^{3}H-CPP binding and spatial learning deficits in aged rats. *Psychobiology.*

Pfaff, D. W., Siva, M. T. and Weiss, J. M. (1971). Telemetered recording of hormone effects on hippocampal neurons. *Science* **172**: 394-395.

Plotsky, P. M. (1987). Regulation of hypophysiotropic factors mediating ACTH secretion. *Ann. NY Acad. Sci.* **512**: 205-217.

Plotsky, P. M. and Vale, W. W. (1984). Hemorrhage-induced secretion of corticotropin-releasing factor-like immunoreactivity into the rat hypophysial portal circulation and its inhibition by glucocorticoids. *Endocrinology* **114**: 164-169.

Plotsky, P. M., Otto, S. and Sapolsky, R. M. (1987). Inhibition of immunoreactive corticotropin-releasing factor into the hypophysial-portal circulation by delayed glucocorticoid feedback. *Endocrinology* **119**: 1126-1130.

Poirier, J., Hess, M., May, P. C. and Finch, C. E. (submitted). Cloning of hippocampal poly(A).RNA sequences that increase after entorhinal cortex lesion in adult rat.

Poirier, J., May, P. C., Osterburg, H. H., Geddes, J., Cotman, C. and Finch, C. E. (1990). Selective alterations of RNA in rat hippocampus after entorhinal cortex lesioning. *Proc. Nat. Acad. Sci. U.S.A.* **87**: 303-307.

Powers, R. E., Walker, L. C., DeSouza, E. B., Vale, W. W., Struble, R. G., Whitehouse, P. J. and Price, D. L. (1987). CRF-like immunoreactivity in the CNS of Alzheimer's disease. *Synapse* **1**: 405-414.

Rapaport, P. A., Allaire, Y., Bourliere, F. and Girard, F. (1964). Reactivite au "stress" et capacite d'adaptation a une situation inhabituelle chez le rat jeune, adulte et age. *Gerontologia* **10**: 20-30.

Ratka, A., Sutanto, W., Bloemers, M., and DeKloet, E. R. (1989). On the role of brain mineralocorticoid (type I). and glucocorticoid (type II) receptors in neuroendocrine regulation. *Neuroendocrinology* **50**: 117-123.

Reul, J. M. H. M. and DeKloet, E. R. (1985). Two receptor systems for corticosterone in rat brain: microdistribution and differential occupation. *Endocrinology* **117**: 2505-2511.

Reul, J. M. H. M. and DeKloet, E. R. (1986). Anatomical resolution of two types of corticosterone receptor sites in the rat brain with *in vitro* autoradiography and computerized image analysis. *J. Steroid Biochem.* **24**: 269-272.

Reul, J. M. H. M., van den Bosch, F. R. and DeKloet, E. R. (1987). Relative occupation of type-I and type-II corticosteroid receptors in rat brain following stress and dexamethasone treatment: functional implications. *J. Endocrinology* **115**: 459-467.

Reul, J. M. H. M., Tonnaer, J. and DeKloet, E. R. (1988). Neurotrophic ACTH analogue promotes plasticity of type I corticosteroid receptors in brain of senescent male rats. *Neurobiol. Aging* **9**: 253-257.

Ritger, H., Veldhuis, H. and DeKloet, E. R. (1984). Spatial orientation and hippocampal corticosterone receptor systems of old rats: Effects of ACTH4-9 analogue ORG2766. *Brain Res.* **309**: 393-399.

Rivier, C. and Vale, W. W. (1983). Effects of angiotensin II on ACTH release *in vivo*: role of corticotropin-releasing factor (CRF). *Regul. Peptides* **7**: 253-258.

Rivier, C. and Plotsky, P. M. (1986). Mediation by corticotropin-releasing factor of adenohypophysial hormone secretion. *Ann. Rev. Physiol.* **48**: 475-489.

Rivier, C., Brownstein, M., Spiess, J., Rivier, J. and Vale, W. (1982). *In vivo* corticotropin-releasing factor-induced secretion of adrenocorticotropin, β-endorphin, and corticosterone. *Endocrinology* **110**: 272-278.

Rowe, J. W. and Kahn, R.L. (1987). Human aging: usual and successful. *Science* **237**: 143-151.

Sapolsky, R. M. (1985a). A mechanism for increased glucocorticoid toxicity in the hippocampus: increased neuronal vulnerability to metabolic insults. *J. Neurosci.* **5**: 1227-1232.

Sapolsky, R. M. (1985b). Glucocorticoid toxicity in the hippocampus: temporal aspects of neuronal vulnerability. *Brain Res.* **359**: 300-307.

Sapolsky, R. M. (1986). Glucocorticoid toxicity in the hippocampus: reversal with supplementation with brain fuels. *J. Neurosci.* **6**: 2240-2245.

Sapolsky, R. M. and Pulsinelli, W. (1985). Glucocorticoids potentiate ischemic injury to neurons: therapeutic implications. *Science* **229**: 1397-1400.

Sapolsky, R. M. and Meaney, M. J. (1986). The maturation of the adrenocortical stress response in the rat. *Brain Res. Rev.* **11**: 65-76.

Sapolsky, R. M. and Meaney, M. J. (1988). Postmortem decay in glucocorticoid binding in human and primate brain. *Brain Res.* **448**: 182-185.

Sapolsky, R. M., Krey, L. C. and McEwen, B. S. (1983a). The adrenocortical response in the aged rat: impairment of recovery from stress. *J. Exptl. Geront.* **18**: 55-63.

Sapolsky, R. M., Krey, L. C. and McEwen, B. S. (1983b). Corticosterone receptors decline in a site-specific manner in the aged rat. *Brain Res.* **289**: 235-240.

Sapolsky, R. M., Krey, L. C. and McEwen, B. S. (1984a). Glucocorticoid-sensitive hippocampal neurons are involved in terminating the adrenocortical stress response. *Proc. Nat. Acad. Sci. U.S.A.* **81**: 6174-6177.

Sapolsky, R. M., Krey, L. C. and McEwen, B. S. (1984b). Stress down-regulated corticosterone receptors in a site-specific manner. *Endocrinology* **114**: 287-292.

Sapolsky, R. M., Krey, L. C. and McEwen, B. S. (1985). Prolonged glucocorticoid exposure reduced hippocampal neuron number: implications for aging. *J. Neurosci.* **5**: 1221-1226.

Sapolsky, R. M., Krey, L. C. and McEwen, B. S. (1986a). The neuroendocrinology of stress and aging: the glucocorticoid cascade hypothesis. *Endo. Rev.* **7**: 284-301.

Sapolsky, R. M., Krey, L. C. and McEwen, B. S. (1986b). The adrenocortical axis in the aged rat: impaired sensitivity to both fast and delayed feedback inhibition. *Neurobiol. Aging* **7**: 331-336.

Sapolsky, R. M., Armanini, M., Packan, D. and Tombaugh, G. (1987). Stress and glucocorticoids in aging. *Endocrinol. Metabol. Clinics* **16**: 965-980.

Sapolsky, R. M., Packan, D. and Vale, W. W. (1988). Glucocorticoid toxicity in the hippocampus: *in vitro* demonstration. *Brain Res.* **453**: 367-374.

Sarrieau, A., Sharma, S. and Meaney, M. J. (1988a). Postnatal development and environmental regulation of hippocampal glucocorticoid and mineralocorticoid receptors in the rat. *Dev. Brain Res.* **43**: 158-162.

Sarrieau, A., Dussaillant, M., Sapolsky, R. M., Aitken, D. H., Olivier, O., Lal, S., Rostene, W. H., Quirion, R. and Meaney, M. J. (1988b). Glucocorticoid binding sites in human temporal cortex. *Brain Res.* **442**: 159-163.

Scheff, S. W. and DeKosky, S. T. (1983). Steroid suppression of axon sprouting in the hippocampal dentate gyrus of the adult rat: dose–response relationship. *Exptl. Neurol.* **82**: 183-191.

Scheff, S. W., Benardo, L. S. and Cotman, C. W. (1980a). Decline in reactive fiber growth in the dentate gyrus of aged rats compared to young adult rats following entorhinal cortex removal. *Brain Res.* **199**: 21-38.

Scheff, S. W., Benardo, L. S. and Cotman, C. W. (1980b). Hydrocortisone administration retards axon sprouting in rat dentate gyrus. *Exptl. Neurol.* **68**: 195-201.

Seisjo, B. (1981). Cell damage in the brain: a speculative synthesis. *J. Cereb. Blood Flow Metabol.* **1**: 155-175.

Selye, H. (1950). *The Physiology and Pathology of Exposure to Stress.*, Acta, Montreal.

Sencar-Cupovic, I. and Milkovic, S. (1976). The development of sex differences in adrenal morphology and responsiveness to stress of rats from birth to end of life. *Mech. Ageing Develop.* **5**: 1-9.

Sharma, M., Palacios-Bois, J., Schwartz, G., Iskandar, H., Thakur, M., Quirion, R. and Nair, N. P. V. (1989). Circadian rhythms of melatonin and cortisol in aging. *Biol. Psychiat.* **25**: 305-319.

Sheppard, K. E. and Funder, J. W. (1987). Equivalent affinity of aldosterone and corticosterone for type I receptors in kidney and hippocampus: direct binding studies. *J. Steroid Biochem.* **28**: 737-742.

Sonntag, W. E., Golieszek, A. G., Brodish, A. and Eldridge, J. C. (1987). Diminished diurnal secretion of adrenocorticotropin (ACTH), but not corticosterone, in old male rats: Possible relation to increased adrenal sensitivity to ACTH *in vivo.* *Endocrinology* **120**: 2308-2315.

Starkman, M. N., Schteingart, D. E. and Schork, M. (1981). Depressed mood and other psychiatric manifestations of Cushing's Syndrome: relationship to hormone levels. *Psychosom. Med.* **43**: 3-18.

Starkman, M. N. and Schteingart, D. E. (1981). Neuropsychiatric manifestations of patients with Cushing's syndrome. *Arch. Internal Med.* **141**: 215-218.

Stern, J. and Levine, S. (1974). Psychobiological aspects of lactation in rats. *Prog. Brain Res.* **41**: 433-444.

Steward, O. and Vincent, S. L. (1983). The process of reinnervation in the dentate gyrus of the adult rat: a quantitative electron microscopic analysis of terminal proliferation and reactive synaptogenesis. *J. Comp. Neurol.* **214**: 370-386.

Steward, O., Torre, E. R., Phillips, L. L. and Trimmer, P. A. (1990). The process of reinnervation in the dentate gyrus of adult rats: time course of increases in mRNA for glial fibrillary acidic protein. *J. Neurosci.* **10**: 2373-2384.

Swanson, L. W., Sawchenko, P. E., Lind, R. W. and Rho, J. H. (1987). The CRH motoneuron: differential peptide regulation in neurons with possible synaptic, paracrine, and endocrine outputs. *Ann. NY Acad. Sci.* **512**: 12-23.

Tang, F. and Philips, J. G. (1978). Some age-related changes in pituitary-adrenal function in the male laboratory rat. *J. Gerontol.* **33**: 377-382.

Tornello, S., Orti, E., DeNicola, A. F., Rainbow, T. C. and McEwen, B. S. (1982). Regulation of glucocorticoid receptors in brain by corticosterone treatment of adrenalectomized rats. *Neuroendocrinology* **35**: 411-417.

Tuszynski, M. D., Buzsaki, G. and Gage, F. H. (1990). Nerve growth factor infusions combined with fetal hippocampal grafts enhance reconstruction of the lesioned septohippocampal projections. *Neurosci.* **36**: 33-44.

Unsicker, K., Kirsch, B., Otten, U. and Thoenen, H. (1978). Nerve growth factor-induced fiber outgrowth from isolated rat arenas chromafin cells: impairment by glucocorticoids. *Proc. Nat. Acad. Sci. U.S.A.* **75**: 3498-3502.

Van Loon, G. R. and DeSouza, E. B. (1987). Regulation of stress-induced secretion of POMC-derived peptides. *Ann. NY Acad. Sci.* **512**: 300-307.

Whelan, T. B., Schteingart, D. E., Starkman, M. N. and Smith, A. (1980). Neuropsychological defects in Cushing's syndrome. *J. Nerv. Mental Dis.* **168**: 753-757.

Wilson, M., Greer, M. and Roberts, L. (1980). Hippocampal inhibition of pituitary-adrenocortical function in female rats. *Brain Res.* **197**: 344-351.

Wrange, O. and Yu, Z.-Y. (1983). Mineralocorticoid receptor in rat kidney and hippocampus: characterization and quantitation by isoelectric focussing. *Endocrinology* **113**: 243-250.

Zarrow, M. X., Campbel, P. S. and Denenberg, V. H. (1972). Handling in infancy: increased levels of the hypothalamic corticotropin releasing factor (CRF) following exposure to a novel situation. *Proc. Soc. Exp. Biol. Med.* **356**: 141-143.

Neuroimmunological Processes and Aging

GEORGE B. STEFANO[1], LISA MALLOZZI[1], STEPHEN PRYOR[1], GREGORY L. FRICCHIONE[2] and THOMAS V. BILFINGER[3]

[1] *Multidisciplinary Center for the Study of Aging, State University of New York, College at Old Westbury, Old Westbury, New York 11568, U.S.A*
[2] *Brigham's Womens Hospital, Division of Psychiatry, Harvard Medical School, Boston, Mass., U.S.A.*
[3] *Department of Surgery, Health Science Center, University Hospital, SUNY at Stony Brook, Stony Brook, NY 11794, U.S.A.*

Introduction

In order to fully understand the implications of age-related alterations or decline in brain function, it is important also to be aware of a growing body of evidence that strongly demonstrates that the nervous and immune systems communicate with each other. This interdependence of the nervous and immune systems is an important consideration for development of active pharmacological interventions for compensation of age-related changes in brain function and in overall health.

Both early Egyptian and Greek civilizations taught that fighting disease was an activity that involved the "mind". Galen, a Greek physician, also noted this apparent interaction in A.D. 200. Today, information concerning the interaction and interdependence of the immune, endocrine and nervous systems is well documented (Blalock, 1989). Anatomical (hard wiring) studies have shown that various immunocompetent tissues are innervated by both sensory and motor neural elements. This has been shown for bone marrow, spleen and thymus (Bullock, 1983). Functional significance of these innervations has been noted when these nerve fibers have been disturbed. Brain lesioning or sympathectomy has the potential for either suppressing or enhancing various immune responses.

Both the nervous and immune systems share many of the same signal molecules (Smith and Blalock, 1981; Blalock, 1989; Stefano, 1989, 1991). These neurotransmitters/modulators are, for example, vasoactive intestinal peptide, adrenocorticotropin (ACTH), and various opioid substances (enkephalin and endorphins). Evidence for neuroimmune and immune autoregulatory mechanisms involving opioid peptides is quite overwhelming. Bioactive neuropeptides, whose multiple roles in the nervous system are well established, are known to affect immunologically competent cells (Smith and Blalock, 1981; review, Blalock, 1989; Stefano, 1989). There is sufficient evidence that these substances, in addition to their interaction with the neuroendocrine apparatus, play a role in autoregulatory immune processes.

In the context of this text devoted to neurobiological aspects of aging, a basic introduction is presented here to familiarize the reader with the cellular components of the immune system. It is hoped that this will provide the reader with sufficient background to be aware of elements of the immune system which have the potential to interact with the nervous system as well as to gain some understanding of how aging may relate to this interaction.

Immune cells can be identified/typed according to their surface "markers" and functions. B-lymphocytes are a type of lymphocyte that originates in bone marrow in mammals. These cells express immunoglobulin both in the cytoplasm and cell surface. B-cells are antibody expressing and producing cells. T-lymphocytes (thymic origin) regulate immune reactions as well as destroy altered "self" cells. Helper cells are so designated because they enhance immune activity/reactions. Other types of T-lymphocytes are cytotoxic and suppressor cells. These cells may liberate and produce immune chemical signal molecules called lymphokines. Examples of lymphokines are interleukin-2 as well as interferon-gamma.

Other important cells for our consideration are the natural killer cells, possibly derived from T-lymphocytes, which may destroy virus-infected cells as well as tumors. Killer cells produce a compound that inhibits virus replication called interferon-alpha. Granulocytes (polymorphonuclear leukocytes) are another class of cells that are involved with phagocytosis of bacteria and damaged "self" cells. Granulocytes are classified as basophils, neutrophils and eosinophils. Lastly, another immune cell type is the monocyte/macrophage. Monocytes may differentiate into macrophages upon stimulation by various signal molecules. A major function of this cell type is phagocytosis. The cell can also produce cytokines (lymphokine) such as interleukin-1. Thus, the cellular immune system contains many different cells that are capable of synergistic as well as antagonistic activities with other cells. This level of complexity again necessitates the existence of complex regulatory loops not only within this system but in its integration with other systems.

Specific immune cells are not only capable of responding to neuropeptides, but also of synthesizing them (Zurawski *et al.*, 1986; Stefano *et al.*, 1989a). Furthermore, chemotactic effects of endogenous opioid peptides on polymorphonuclear leukocytes, monocytes, and lymphocytes have been demonstrated (Brown *et al.*, 1986; Falke and Fischer, 1985; Fischer and Falke, 1984, 1986; Stefano *et al.*, 1989a, b). Opioid substances have thus been shown to have diverse functions that transcend their originally proposed role in nociceptive/analgesic systems (Stefano, 1982; Leung and Stefano, 1987). The importance of this family of compounds is highlighted even more by the discovery of their occurrence in invertebrates. Moreover, Stefano *et al.* (1989a, b) have demonstrated that opioids, by stereoselective mechanisms, are involved in invertebrate immune mechanisms.

This chapter will attempt to document that the opioid-immune relationship found in mammals is comparable to that in invertebrates. Additionally, given the extensiveness of this system in immunomodulation, its potential significance in the aging process is discussed.

The immune system and age-related phenomena

The immune system can be conceived as capable of establishing and/or maintaining internal homeostasis by modifying various physiological processes, especially those under neural control, when confronted with assaults on "self" and "non-self". Both antibody and precise cellular proliferation mechanisms, which are at the center of an immune response, are so sophisticated that they require precise, select and absolute regulatory mechanisms. Clearly, the immune systems of all animals must recognize non-self tissues and cells and protect the organism from noncognitive and cognitive assaults within its realm of functional capabilities. In this regard, cellular and humoral immune responses are of vital importance. It would seem that through the course of evolution a successful "immune" plan had to be developed and maintained regardless of the degree of complexity of the organism that expresses it. This "protective" function can be regarded as an important factor in extending the quality of life as well as providing for longevity.

Aging affects the immune system in many ways. Although not every aged individual exhibits a decline in all immune functions, on a population level nearly every immune function declines with age. Age-associated immune system changes have been studied in both experimental animals and humans. There are four basic areas of immune senescence that have been examined: thymic involution, age-associated changes in lymphocytes, age-associated changes in humoral immunity and age-associated changes in cell mediated immunity.

Thymus involution

The involution of the thymus gland with age has long been noted in both humans and experimental animals (Boyd, 1932; Andrew, 1952). The thymus gland reaches its maximum at sexual maturity in humans then gradually shrinks, reaching only 5% to 10% of its original size by age 45 (Hirokawa and Makinodan, 1975). The thymus is both an important endocrine organ for immunity and a site of immune cell differentiation. Both of these functions are affected by thymic involution. Serum levels of thymic hormones, important in the differentiation of pre- and post-thymic lymphocytes, fall between the ages of 20 and 30, and can no longer be detected after 60 years of age (Lewis *et al.*, 1978). The differentiation of immature lymphoid cells from the bone marrow is impeded as the thymus gland involutes with age. This suggests that the thymus loses its capacity to cause differentiation.

One aspect of maturation of lymphoid cells in human thymus is the acquisition of surface receptors for sheep erythrocytes which declines with age from 95% under 20 years to about 50% at 60 years of age or greater (Singh and Singh, 1979). Another indication of differentiation is the percent of T-lymphocytes which bind autologous erythrocytes forming rosettes. Only immature lymphocytes bind autologous erythrocytes and their number in the blood increases with age (Moody *et al.*, 1981; Fournier and Charreire, 1981). Thus, thymic involution is associated with a decrease in the serum thymic hormone, and an increased number of immature T-lymphocytes in the thymus and in the peripheral blood.

Experiments with young lethally irradiated, thymectomized mice have shown that the age of the thymus tissue may affect its function (Hirokawa and Makinodan, 1975). The aging and involution of the thymus also affects humoral immunity indirectly through the regulatory activity of helper and suppressor T-lymphocytes. It also directly influences the maturation of B-lymphocytes. Thymus gland transplant studies show that the capacity to generate a heterologous immune response with respect to affinity by B-cells is less in thymus transplants from older animals (Siskind *et al.*, 1981; Szewczuk and Campbell, 1980; Sherr *et al.*, 1978).

Age associated changes in lymphocytes

The total number of lymphocytes and the number of T- and B-lymphocytes in the peripheral blood of man and experimental animals do not change appreciably with age. However, there is a change in the proportion of cell subpopulations. As we have seen, there is an age-associated increase in immature T-lymphocytes that form rosettes with autologous erythrocytes in human and experimental animals. There is also an increase in T-gamma-lymphocytes with age in humans. There also appears to be an age-associated shift in the proportion of various lymphocyte subtypes. In expression of the cell surface glycoprotein CD8 and CD4, some groups report increases of CD4 (Moody *et al.*, 1981; Bender *et al.*, 1988) and others of CD8 cells (Thompson *et al.*, 1984), whereas others report no change (Rabinowe *et al.*, 1987). Using a different antibody, Rabinowe *et al.* (1987) have found a 58% increase in 3G5 marker on T-lymphocytes with age. Utsuyama and Hirokawa (1987) report a change from CD8 bright to CD8 dim cells with age. Additionally, Lerner *et al*, (1989) have found higher numbers of cells with the marker PGP-1 in older organisms.

New cell surface determinants on lymphocytes may arise with age. Novel antigens may be expressed by lymphocytes from aged animals which are recognized by young syngeneic mice (Callard *et al.*, 1979). The density of some receptors also change with age. The theta determinant and the receptor for T-cell growth factor on the surface of T-cells declines with age, as does the density of surface immunoglobulin on B-cells (Brennan and Jaroslow, 1975; Thoman and Weigle, 1981; Rosenberg *et al*, 1982; Woda and Feldman, 1979). These alternations of surface receptors may reflect a change in the membrane composition and cytoskeleton of aged animals. Capping of membrane proteins is closely related to the lateral mobility of glycoproteins in the lipid bilayer (Schreiner *et al.*, 1977). This may reflect changes in the viscosity of the bilayer due to an increase in the molar ratio of cholesterol to phospholipids with age (Rivany *et al.*, 1979).

Enzymes found in lymphocytes also change with age. Lymphocyte adenylate cyclase in experimental animals increases with age while guanylate cyclase decreases. Paradoxically, the content of cyclic AMP decreases and cyclic GMP increases with age (Tam and Walford, 1978, 1980). Purine nucleoside phosphorylase has been found to decrease with age concomitantly with a decline in T-cell function (Scholar *et al.*, 1980). DNA repair enzymes may also decline in function as evidenced by the increased susceptibility of lymphocytes from the aged to ionizing radiation, ultraviolet light and mutagenic drugs (Lambert *et al.*, 1977; Seshadri *et al.*, 1979; Walford and Bergman, 1979).

Humoral immunity

Another major aspect of the immune system that exhibits change with age is humoral immunity. There appears to be a small, but statistically significant, change in the concentration of immunoglobulins in the blood serum with age. IgA and IgG antibodies in human serum increase with age and IgM antibodies decrease. IgA and IgG also appear to increase in cerebrospinal fluid of older humans (Radl *et al.*, 1975; Buckley and Dorsey, 1970; Nerenberg and Prasod, 1975). There is also a decline in the ability of mice and humans to mount an IgE response to antigen challenge (Fujiwara and Kishimoto, 1979).

Two significant changes in humoral immunity with age are the decrease in concentration of natural antibodies and the rise in concentrations of autoantibodies in blood serum (Paul and Bunnell, 1932; Thomsen and Kettel, 1929; Hallgren and Yunis, 1980; Rowley *et al.*, 1968; Pandey *et al.*, 1979; Cammarata *et al.*, 1967). This decline in natural antibodies and rise in autoantibodies may contribute to the deregulation of the immune system. An important class of autoantibodies is the auto-anti idiotypic antibodies involved in down-regulation of the immune response. Excessive amounts of auto-anti-idiotypic antibody are expressed by old experimental animals during the immune response (Goidl *et al.*, 1980; Szewczuk and Campbell, 1980). Auto-anti-idiotypic antibodies block lymphocyte secretion of specific antibody. Hence, the excessive amounts of these antibodies may not only reflect immune decline but actually contribute to the senescence of the immune system, including the loss of self tolerance noted in aged individuals. This possibility is also suggested by experiments with syngeneic mice that show that injected lymphocytes from old animals can induce graft versus host rejection (Gozes *et al.*, 1978). The induction of B-lymphocyte and T-lymphocyte tolerance to exogenous antigens in autoimmune mice is also much more difficult in aged animals (Dobken *et al.*, 1980).

Monoclonal immunoglobulins increase with age (Radl *et al.*, 1975; Axelsson *et al.*, 1966). These homogeneous immune proteins may be due to a disordered immune regulation of normal B lymphocytes. Below the age of 50, less than 0.1% of humans have monoclonal immunoglobulins in their serum while 2% over 70 years of age have them. Mice also show a rise in the incidence of monoclonal antibodies with age (Radl, 1980).

The response of humans and experimental animals to foreign antigens decreases with age (Roberts-Thomson *et al.*, 1974; Ammann *et al.*, 1980; Kishimoto *et al.*, 1976; Whittingham *et al.*, 1978). The antibody response to Japanese B encephalitis and parainfluenza also decreases with age in humans (Sabin *et al.*, 1947). Studies with experimental animals that reveal peak antibody responses are usually observed during the first third of the life span and then decline. The primary response is usually more compromised with age than the secondary (Makinodan and Peterson, 1962; Makinodan and Adler, 1975). Perhaps one of the most important changes seen in humoral immunity with age comes from a change in the number and function of T-helper lymphocytes in relation to T-suppressor lymphocytes. This has been documented in cell transfer studies and *in vitro* studies of immune response (Goidl *et al.*, 1976; Dekruyff *et al.*, 1980a; Kim *et al.*, 1982; Nagel *et al.*, 1981). The decline in function of these cells is apparently intrinsic to the cell rather than being merely a function of the environment within an elderly host. This is illustrated experimentally by the transfer of lymphocytes from old mice to young syngeneic, thymectomized lethally irradiated young mice. Old helper T-lymphocytes displayed the same reduced response to foreign antigens with a preferential loss of high affinity and IgG antibodies as lymphocytes in old animals. However, if the thymus of the young animal recipients was left intact, or if young thymocytes were injected with old lymphocytes, then immune response of the old T-lymphocyte was greatly improved. The immune response was also improved by injection of thymopoietin or *in vitro* incubation of the old T-lymphocytes in thymic hormone before transfer (Goidl *et al.*, 1976; Dekruyff *et al.*, 1980a; Callard *et al.*, 1979, 1980). *In vitro* studies of antibody secretions in human lymphocytes confirm that the major defect in old lymphocytes is due to impaired T lymphocyte function. In these preparations there appears to be a deficiency of helper T-cells and/or increase in suppressor T-cell activity with age.

In contrast to T-cell function, other immune cells involved in humoral immunity do not generally decline with age in humans or experimental animals. In B-cells, the proliferative response induced by anti-immunoglobulin antibody does not decline with age (Weiner *et al.*, 1978). The proliferative response of B-cells to lypopolysaccharide is not significantly impaired with age (Kishimoto *et al.*, 1976; Ammann *et al.*, 1980; Gerbase-Delima *et al.*, 1975). Macrophage function also is not significantly affected by age (Kim *et al.*, 1982; Gardner *et al.*, 1981).

Cell-mediated immunity

Cell-mediated immunity is primarily a function of the thymic dependent lymphocytes and has been noted to decline with the involution of the thymus. Several studies have related the senescence of cell-mediated immunity to the functional capacity of T-lymphocytes from individuals of different ages. Two measures of cell-mediated immunity commonly used *in vivo* are delayed hypersensitivity and graft rejection. Elderly people generally have less vigorous delayed hypersensitive reactions to antigens such as *Candida* and mumps than younger people (Roberts-Thompson *et al.*, 1974). This may be due to a loss of immunological memory or altered response to antigenic challenge or both. Apparently the difference in time between sensitization and subsequent challenge is not a factor since old individuals fail to respond to a new antigen in greater frequency than younger individuals, even when the response interval was the same (Walford *et al.*, 1968).

Graft versus host experiments in animals also illustrate a decline in cell-mediated immunity with age. Graft rejection is the response of an integrated series of immune reactions including antigen recognition and display, helper T-lymphocyte proliferation, and the generation of cytotoxic T-lymphocytes. It is the cytotoxic T-cells along with natural killer cells that are the effectors of graft rejection. Older mice have an impaired ability to reject tissue and tumor grafts. There appears to be an age-related decrease in both the number of cytotoxic T-cells and in their functional potencies against tumor cells in mice (Zharhary and Gershon, 1981). The number of natural killer cells and the ability of these cells to lyse tumors also declines in older mice (Roder, 1975). However, the number and natural killer activity of natural killer cells does not appear to decline with age in humans, nor does the interferon-inducible natural killer activity of lymphocytes seem to diminish (Fernandes and Gupta, 1981).

Cell-mediated immunity is also responsible for resistance to viral infections. T-cell-mediated immunity to *Listeria monocytogenes* has been shown to decline with age in mice. Old infected mice developed only one thousandth the level of T-cell immunity as young infected mice (Patel, 1981). In general, old mice show a delayed generation of cytotoxic T-lymphocytes, a lower peak cytotoxic response, and a shorter duration of cytotoxic activity (Doherty, 1977; Patel, 1981).

Another aspect of cell-mediated immune dysfunction with age is the presence of autoimmune T-lymphocytes in old animals. Lymphocytes transferred from old animals to young syngeneic recipients may cause a graft versus host response to tissue of the same genotype. This reaction does not occur in younger syngeneic lymphocyte transfers. This may be indicative that the increase in autoimmune response seen in older animals is a manifestation of cell-mediated as well as humoral-mediated immunity.

Summary

There are many changes in the immune system with age that may account for both the decrease in resistance to infection and other pathology associated with aging. Both humoral and cell-mediated response to foreign antigens declines with age, while the response to one's own antigens increases. These immune changes are related to a shrinking of the thymus gland, alterations in the number and function of T-cell subsets, and a shift from idiotypic to anti-idiotypic activity. A decline in immune surveillance may be related to neoplastic diseases and perhaps to cardiovascular disease. The immune reaction to self may contribute to damaged tissues and organs and other pathological manifestations of aging.

Neuroimmunology and aging

Modulation of immunoresponsive mammalian and invertebrate cells

A functional characteristic of polymorphonuclear leukocytes (PMN), lymphocytes and monocytes is chemotaxis, the directional movement of cells responding to a chemical gradient. A major mechanism responsible for the accumulation of PMN, monocytes, or lymphocytes at sites of inflammation or antigenic challenge is the activity of chemotactic factors. Chemotactic stimuli seem to be responsible for the type of immunocompetent cell that accumulates at an inflammatory site, that is, cell-specific signal molecules may perform this function along with their respective stereospecific receptors. Chemotaxis is in all likelihood one of the most critical immune phenomena in that it enables mobile cells to accumulate at sites of inflammation or antigenic challenge.

Evidence for a chemotactic role for opioids can be obtained in mammals by intraventricular injections of beta-endorphin or Met-enkephalin which result in the appearance of macrophage-like cells in the cerebrospinal fluid (Saland *et al.,* 1983; Van Epps *et al.,* 1983a, b). These data support a chemotactic function being mediated, at least in part, by various opioid peptides.

Along with the stimulating effect of opioids on migratory behavior comes that of cellular adherence. Opioid peptides were found to enhance adherence of neutrophils in a naloxone reversible manner (Brown *et al.,* 1986; Stefano *et al.,* 1989a). Interestingly, the dose-dependent effect is bimodal, as noted earlier in reference to the migratory activity of these cells.

It has also been observed that beta-endorphin induces PMNs to increase their diameter by approximately 20% in at least 33% of the total cellular population examined (Falke and Fischer, 1985). This increase in size is primarily due to cellular elongation. This phenomenon cannot be observed in rat and dog PMN, but is seen in rabbit and very pronounced in human cells (Falke and Fischer, 1985; Stefano, 1989). It has recently been demonstrated that human leukocytes increase their area by flattening and then become mobile when stimulated with DAMA (Stefano *et al.*, 1989b). The more rounded ("inactive") cells exhibit a locomotory response and increase their velocity in the presence of beta-endorphin as compared with that of nontreated controls (Fischer and Falke, 1986). The results of these studies indicate that opioids participate in the initial phase of an immune response by initiating adherence as well as cellular motility.

A subpopulation of immunocytes of *Mytilus edulis* and *Leucophaea maderae* have the ability to respond to low opioid concentrations by adhering and clumping (Stefano *et al.*, 1989a). Exogenous Met-enkephalin did not increase cellular adherence above control levels at low doses, due to the presence of proteolytic enzymes, specifically neutral endopeptidase 24.11 (Shipp *et al.*,. 1990). *Mytilus* immunocytes upon the presentation of DAMA also undergo conformational changes indicative of "activation" as a prelude to locomotion (Stefano *et al.*, 1989b).

In a T-helper cell line from a Con A-stimulated mouse an open reading frame was discovered that contained 93% homology with rat brain preproenkephalin mRNA (Zurawski *et al.*, 1986). This sequence was only made evident by mitogen stimulation. The cells that produced this mRNA appeared to secrete immunoreactive Met-enkephalin. Smith *et al.*, (1986) found immunoreactive beta-endorphin in supernatants of human peripheral blood lymphocytes following corticotropin-releasing factor treatments. Immunoreactive beta-endorphin has been detected in plasma cells of canine colon (Grube, 1980), and Met-enkephalin in splenic white pulp of the rat (Felten *et al.*, 1985). The presence of opioid peptides in cell-free hemolymph and hemocytes, respectively, of *Mytilus* was demonstrated by Stefano *et al.*, (1989a). Since it would appear that "free" enkephalin-like material is present in the hemolymph, we can surmise that mechanisms exist to protect it from proteolytic degradation. These phenomena should be taken into consideration in future studies of the effects of opioid drugs and their mode of operation in immunoregulation.

Signal transduction mechanisms

Studies of neuroimmunology and aging have focused on cellular communication in regard to lymphokine production. Many groups have documented an age-related decline in the production of interleukin-2 (IL-2), a B- and T-cell growth factor (Gillis *et al.*, 1981; Nagel *et al.*, 1988) associated with a decline of target cell responsiveness to the factor (Thoman and Weigle, 1982, 1985). Nagel *et al.*, (1988) have demonstrated a decline in the number of cells that express IL-2 receptors. Indeed, Wu *et al.*, (1986) have shown declines of IL-2 mRNA in old rats and humans (Nagel *et al.*, 1988). In general, the data seem to indicate that T-cells are present in older organisms but they contain greater numbers of cells that do not respond to known activators.

In normal T-cells and granulocytes following Con A (mitogen) administration, cells display an increase in intracellular calcium. In aged cells, however, the proportion of cells that exhibit this activation spike is reduced (Miller *et al.*, 1987; Lipschitz *et al.*, 1988). Thus, there appears to be a failure in the signal transduction mechanism within the cell that is responsible for the decrease in unresponsive cells. Notably, this work is relatively new and must await future studies to determine its significance.

Aging and autoimmunoregulatory processes

Age-related changes in the involvement of opioid neuropeptides in immunoregulatory processes were studied in human blood as well as hemolymph of the mollusc *Mytilus edulis* (Stefano *et al.*, 1991). In human blood serum the levels of circulating Met-enkephalin-like material were found to rise with increasing age of the donors, and to decrease drastically near the end of their expected potential life expectancy (80-92 years). The same changes occurred in *Mytilus* examined at the estimated ages of 1-2 to 5-6 years. In addition, both groups showed a significant age-related difference with respect to the cellular responses to opioid challenge. In blood from human donors (ages 25-59), 30-35% of the granulocytes responded to the administration of the Met-enkephalin analog D-Ala^2-Met^5-enkephalinamide by showing conformational changes indicative of stimulation and increased locomotory activity. By contrast, specimens of donors aged 60-79 years yielded the same responses in only 20% of the population. A comparable decrease in cellular response was observed in hemolymph from *Mytilus* observed at young and older ages (32-36% in young and 22% in old). Indeed, these results may lead one to surmise that the higher opioid levels associated with aging may "desensitize" immunocyte responsiveness. However, this conclusion is premature.

Recently, cold saturation experiments with the radioligand ^{3}H-(D-Ala^2) deltorphin I and ^{3}H-DAMA revealed the presence of two high affinity delta binding sites on human granulocytes, one sensitive to the non-equilibrium delta opioid antagonist D-Ala^2-Leu^5-Cys^6-enkaphalinamide and the other relatively insensitive. The results obtained with (D-Ala^2) deltorphin I support the view that the special role played by endogenous Met-enkephalin in immunobiological activities of vertebrates and invertebrates is mediated by a special subtype of delta opioid receptor. The potential for this finding to impact on aging studies has yet to be realized, but it offers an interesting level of opioid complexity.

An immune-neuro-link: macrophages potential for age-associted alterations

In a recent review, Stefano and colleagues (1993) discuss the potential for the macrophage to cause neural dysfunction. Briefly, monocytes/macrophages, originating from bone marrow, appear to wander in the circulatory system for a relatively short time before they "settle" in various tissues, such as the central nervous system, as resident microglia. Microglial functions and behavior are not well delineated. However, when cells die in the natural course of CNS development, macrophages can be observed to phagocytize these cells. The macrophage also has potential to secrete neuroactive signal molecules (e.g., interleukin-1 and tumor necrosis factor; see Stefano *et al.*, 1993). An important functional property of mobile immune cells is their migratory behavior toward sites of inflammation or antigenic challenge. They reach their destinations guided (chemotaxis) by concentration gradients of specific signal substances. Chemotaxis is important, since it ensures that cells get to the antigenic challenge. Is chemokinesis, a random non-directed cellular migratory path, just as important in responding to antigenic challenge? We believe the answer is yes. Once a macrophage, for example, arrives at an inflammatory site liberating the chemotaxic stimulus, it must remain there, to perform its functions (phagocytosis, nitric oxide [NO] generation, wound debriding, etc.). We surmise chemokinesis generates macrophage retention through the presence of numerous and highly concentrated signal molecules at the site of antigenic challenge. Chemotaxis and chemokinesis may be the same activity, but the immediate environment (low or high levels of one or more signal molecules) dictates which cellular behavior pattern emerges. It can also be surmised that normal stimuli, inappropriately present (due to trauma, nonspecific synthesis and/or release of chemical signals, viral interaction; see Stefano *et al.*, 1993), may initiate either chemotaxis or chemokinesis. Under these abnormal circumstances, however, the predominant cellular behavior that may emerge is chemokinesis due to the nonspecific stimuli and the potential for the macrophage, once activated, to produce numerous secretory products. Under abnormal stimulation it is possible that the macrophages, due to nonspecific "hyperstimulation", may become unable to respond to normal antigenic challenge and are thereby "immunosuppressed" or simply dysfunctional. Given the numerous macrophage secretory products, in this immunosuppressed-hyperstimulated state, this cell may produce such excessive amounts of these products as to render them toxic. The authors in the review link the macrophage to postcardiotomy delirium, delirium associated with AIDS, as well as the potential of this cell to be involved in other neurological abnormalities. The timeliness of this hypothesis involving immunocytes in neurological disorders has been noted by McGeer and colleagues (1990). In their report it is surmised that the macrophages may play a role in Alzheimer's disease, in that they are found in abundance in damaged neural areas.

Conclusions

A major recent advance in the analysis of the diverse roles played by neuropeptides in intercellular communication concerns their involvement in immunoregulatory processes. Comparable regulatory phenomena also occur in the immune system of invertebrates, as noted in this chapter. Both the invertebrate and vertebrate data imply that the proportion of cells that have the potential to respond to the various signal molecules is rather small and that this population decreases with aging even more.

Recent research concerning neuroimmune mechanisms suggests that it may be possible to utilize immune cells to assess neurological function and stress (Blalock, 1989; Stefano, 1989). Clearly, the neuroimmune and autoimmunoregulatory responsiveness to various signal molecules may well provide a "window" into the physiological and mental state of an organism. Additionally, the information derived from such studies may be useful for the development of patient care and pharmacological treatments, not only for the elderly, but also for individuals suffering from certain organic and/or psychiatric disorders.

Acknowledgements

The authors wish to thank the many collaborators and students that worked on the various projects outlined in this review. During the preparation of the manuscript the authors were partially supported by NIH-MBRS MH-08180, ADAMHA-MARC 17138, NSF INT-8803664 and ADAMHA-47392 and the State University of New York Research Foundation.

References

Ammann, A. J., Schiffman, G. and Austrian, R. (1980).The antibody responses to pneumococcal capsular polysaccharides in aged individuals. *Proc. Soc. Exp. Biol. Med.* **164**: 312-316.

Andrew, W. (1952). In: *Cellular Changes with Age*, Springfield, III: Charles C. Thomas. pp. 3-74.

Axelsson, U., Bachmann, R. and Hallen, J. (1966). Frequency of pathological proteins (M-components) in 6,995 sera from an adult population. *Acta Medica Scandinavica* **179**: 235-246.

Bender, B. S., Chrest, F. J., Nagel, J. A. and Adler, W. H. (1988). Peripheral blood CD8+ subsets in young and elderly adults: enumeration by two-color immunofluorescence and flow cytometry. *Aging: Immunol. Infect. Dis.* **1**: 23-30.

Blalock, J. E. (1989). A molecular basis for bidirectional communication between the immune and neuroendocrine systems. *Physiol. Rev.* **69**: 1-32.

Boyd, E. (1932). The weight of the thymus gland in health and in disease. *Amer. J. Dis. Child* **43**: 1162-1214.

Brennan, P. C. and Jaroslow, B. N. (1975). Age-associated decline in theta antigen on spleen thymus-derived lymphocytes of B6CF mice. *Cell. Immunol.* **15**: 51-56.

Brown, S. L., Tokuda, S., Saland, L. C., and Van Epps, D. E., (1986). Opioid peptides effects on leukocyte migration. In: *Enkephalins and Endorphins: Stress and the Immune System*, eds., N. P. Plotnikoff, R. E. Faith, A. J. Murgo and R. Good, Plenum Press, N.Y. pp. 367-386.

Buckley, C. E. and Dorsey, F. C. (1970). The input of aging on human serum immunoglobulin concentrations. *J. Immunol.* **105**: 964-972.

Bullock, K. (1983). Neuroanatomy of lymphoid tissues: A review In: *Neural Modulation of Immunity*, eds., R. Sullemih, M. Cohn and T. Melnechuk, Raven Press, NY, pp. 111-141.

Callard, R. E., Basten, A. and Blanden, R. V. (1979). Loss of immune competence with age may be due to a qualitative abnormality in lymphocyte membranes. *Nature* **282**: 218-219.

Callard, R. E., Fazekas De St. Groth, B., Basten, A. and McKenzie, I. F. C. (1980). Immune function in aged mice. V. Role of suppressor cells. *J. Immunol.* **124**: 52-58.

Cammarata, R. J., Rodnan, G. P. and Fennell, R. H. (1967). Serum anti-gamma-globulin and antinuclear factors in the aged. *J. Am. Med. Assoc.* **199**: 455-465.

Dekruyff, R. H., Kim, Y. T., Siskind, G. W. and Weksler, M. E. (1980a). Age-related changes in the *in vitro* immune response: increased suppressor activity in immature and aged mice. *J. Immunol.* **125**: 142-147.

Dobken, J., Weksler, M. E. and Siskind, G. W. (1980). Effect of age on ease of B cell tolerance induction. *Cell. Immunol.* **55**: 66-73.

Doherty, P. C. (1977). Diminished T cell surveillance function in old mice infected with lymphocyte choriomeningitis virus. *Immunology* **32**: 751-754.

Falke, N. E. and Fischer, E. G. (1985). Cell shape of polymorphonuclear leukocytes is influenced by opioids. *Immunobiol.* **169**: 532-539.

Felten, D. L., Selten, S. Y., Carlson, S. L., Olschowka, J. A. and Livnat, S. (1985). Noradrenergic and peptidergic innervation of lymphoid tissue. *J. Immunol.* **135**: 755-761.

Fernandes, G. and Gupta, S. (1981). Natural killing and antibody-dependent cytotoxicity by lymphocyte sub-populations in young and aging humans. *J. Clin. Immunol.* **1**: 141-147.

Fischer, E. G. and Falke, N. E. (1984). B-endorphin modulates immune functions – A review. *Psychother. Psychosom.* **42**: 195-204.

Fischer, E. G. and Falke, N. E. (1986). The influence of endogenous opioid peptides on venous granulocytes. In: *Enkephalins and Endorphins: Stress and the Immune System*, eds., N. P. Plotnikoff, R. E. Faith, A. J. Murgo and R. Good, Plenum Press, N.Y. pp. 263-270.

Fournier, C. and Charreire, J. (1981). Autologous mixed lymphocyte reaction in man. I. Relationship with age and sex. *Cell. Immunol.* **60**: 212-219.

Fujiwara, M. and Kishimoto, S. (1979). IgE antibody formation and aging. I. Age-related changes in IgE antibody formation and avidity for the DNP determinant in mice. *J. Immunol.* **123**: 263-268.

Gardner, N. D., Lim, S. T. K. and Lawton, J. W. M. (1981). Monocyte function in ageing humans. *Mech. Ageing Dev.* **16**: 233-239.

Gerbase-Delima, M., Meredith, P. and Walford, R. L. (1975). Age-related changes, including synergy and suppression in the mixed lymphocyte reaction in long-lived mice. *Fed. Proc.* **34**: 159-161.

Gillis, A., Kozak, R., Durante, M. and Weksler, M. E. (1981). Immunological studies of aging. Decreased production of and response to T cell growth factor by lymphocytes from aged humans. *J. Clin. Invest.* **67**: 937-942.

Goidl, E. A., Innes, J. B. and Weksler, M. E. (1976). Immunological studies of aging. II. Loss of IgG and high avidity plaque-forming cells and increased suppressor cell activity in aging mice. *J. Exp. Med.* **144**: 1037-1048.

Goidl, E. A., Thorbeck, G. J., Weksler, M. E. and Siskind, G. W. (1980). Production of auto-anti-idiotypic antibody during the normal immune response: changes in the auto-anti-idiotypic antibody response and the idiotypic repertoire associated with aging. *Proc. Natl. Acad. Sci. USA* **77**: 6788-6792.

Gozes, Y., Umiel, T., Asher, M. and Trainin, N. (1978). Syngeneic GvH induced in popliteal lymph nodes by spleen cells of old C57BL/6 mice. *J. Immunol.* **121**: 2199-2204.

Grube, D. (1980). Alpha-endorphin-like immunoreactivity in plasma cells of the canine colonic mucosa. *Histochemistry* **69**: 157-160.

Hallgren, H. M. and Yunis, E. J. (1980). In: *Immunological aspects of aging*, eds., D. Segre and L. Smith, New York: Marcel Dekker. pp. 281-293.

Hirokawa, K. and Makinodan, T. (1975). Thymic involution: effect on T cell differentiation. *J. Immunol.* **6**: 1659-1664.

Kim, Y. T., Siskind, G. W. and Weksler, M. E. (1982). Cellular basis of the impaired immune response of elderly humans. In: *Human B Lymphocyte Function: Activation and Immunoregulation*, eds., A. S. Fauci and R. E. Ballieux, Raven Press, N.Y., pp. 129-139.

Kishimoto, S., Takahama, T. and Mizumachi, H. (1976). *In vitro* immune response to the 2,4,6-trinitrophenyl determinant in aged C57BL mice: changes in the humoral response to avidity for the TNP determinant and responsiveness to LPS effect with aging. *J. Immunol.* **116**: 294-300.

Lambert, B., Ringbord, N. and Swanbert, B. (1977). Repair on UV-induced DNA lesions in peripheral lymphocytes from healthy subjects of various ages, individuals with Down's syndrome and patients with actinic keratosis. *Mut. Res.* **46**: 133-134.

Lerner, A., Philosophe, B. and Miller, R. A. (1989). Defective calcium in flux and preserved inositol phosphate generation in T cells from old mice. *Aging*: *Immunol. Infect. Dis.* **1**: 149-157.

Leung, M. K. and Stefano, G. B. (1987). Comparative neurobiology of opioids in invertebrates with special attention to senescent alterations. *Progress in Neurobiology* **28**: 131-159.

Lewis, V. M., Twomey, J. J., Bealmear, P., Goldstein, G. and Good, R. A. (1978). Age, thymic involution and circulating thymic hormone activity. *J. Clin. Endocrin. Metabol.* **47**: 145-150.

Lipshitz, D. A., Udupa, K. B. and Boxer, L. A. (1988). The role of calcium in the age-related decline of neutrophil function. *Blood* **71**: 659-665.

Makinodan, T. and Adler, W. H. (1975). Effects of aging on the differentiation and proliferative potentials of cells of the immune system. *Fed. Proc.* **34**: 153-158.

Makinodan, T. and Peterson, W. J. (1962). Relative antibody forming capacity of spleen cells as a function of age. *Proc. Natl. Acad. Sci. USA* **48**: 234-241.

McGeer, P. L., McGeer, E. S., Akiyama, H., Itagaki, S., Harrop, R. and Peppard, R. (1990). Neuronal degeneration and memory loss in Alzheimer's disease and aging. *Exp. Brain Res.* **21**: 411-426.

Miller, R. A., Jacobson, B. and Simons, E. R. (1987). Diminished calcium influx in lectin-stimulated T cells from old mice. *J. Cell Physiol.* **132**: 337-342.

Moody, C. E., Ubbes, J. B., Staiano-Coico, L., Incefy, G. S., Thaler, H. T. and Weksler, M. E. (1981). Lymphocyte transformation induced by autologous cells. XI. The effect of age on the autologous mixed lymphocyte reaction. *J. Immunology* **44**: 431-438.

Nagel, J. A., Chrest, F. J. and Adler, W. H. (1981). Enumeration of T lymphocyte subsets by monoclonal antibodies in young and aged humans. *J. Immunol.* **127**: 2086-2088.

Nagel, J. E., Chopra, R. K., Chrest, F. J., McCoy, M. T., Schneider, E. L., Holbrook, N. J. and Adler, W. H. (1988). Decreased proliferation, interleukin 2 synthesis, and receptor expression are accompanied by decreased mRNA expression in phytohemagglutinin-stimulated cells from elderly donors. *J. Clin. Invest.* **81**: 1096-1102.

Nerenberg, S. T. and Prasod, R. (1975). Radioimmunoassays for Ig classes G, A, M, D and E in spinal fluids: normal values of different age groups. *J. Lab. Clin. Med.* **86**: 887-898.

Pandey, J. P., Fudenberg, H. H., Ainsworth, S. K. and Loadholt, C. B. (1979). Autoantibodies in healthy subjects of different age groups. *Mech. Ageing Dev.* **10**: 399-404.

Patel, P. J. (1981). Aging and antimicrobial immunity. *J. Exp. Med.* **154**: 821-831.

Paul, J. R. and Bunnell, W. W. (1932). Anti-SRBC agglutinin with age. *Am. J. Med. Sci.* **183**: 90-121.

Rabinowe, S. L., Nayak, R. C., Krisch, K., Geroge, K. L. and Eisenbarth, G. S. (1987). Aging in man. Linear increase of novel T cell subset defined by antiganglioside monoclonal antibody 3G5. *J. Exp. Med.* **165**: 1436-1441.

Radl, J., DeGlopper, E., Vanderberg, P. and Van-Zwieten, M. J. (1980). Idiopathic paraproteinemia. III. Increased frequency of rare proteinemia in thymectomized aging C57BL/KaLwRij and CBA/BrARij mice. *J. Immunol.* **125**: 31-35.

Radl, J., Spers, J. M., Skuaril, F., Morell, A. and Hijmans, W. (1975). Immunoglobulin patterns in humans over 95 years of age. *Clin. Exp. Immunol.* **22**: 84-90.

Rivany, B., Globerson, A. and Shiritzky, M. (1979). Viscosity of lymphocyte plasma membrane in aging mice and the possible relation to serum cholesterol. *Mech. Ageing Dev.* **10**: 71-79.

Roberts-Thomson, I. C., Whittingham, S., Youngchaiyud, U. and Mackay, I. R. (1974). Ageing, immune response, and mortality. *Lancet* **2**: 368-370.

Roder, J. C. (1975). Target–effector interaction in the natural killer (NK) cell system. VI. The influence of age and genotype on NK binding characteristics. *Immunol.* **41**: 483-489.

Rosenberg, J. S., Gilman, S. C. and Feldman, J. D. (1982). Activation of rat B lymphocytes. II. Functional and structural changes in "aged" rat B lymphocytes. *J. Immunol.* **128**: 656-660.

Rowley, M. J., Buchanan, H. and MacKay, I. R. (1968). Reciprocal change with age in antibody to extrinisic and intrinsic antigens. *Lancet* **2**: 24-26.

Sabin, A. B., Ginder, D. R., Matumoto, M. and Schlesinger, R. W. (1947). Serological response of Japanese children to Japanese B encephalitis mouse brain vaccine. *Proc. Soc. Exp. Biol. Med.* **67**: 135-140.

Saland, L. C., Van Epps, D. E., Ortiz, E. and Samora, A. (1983). Acute injections of opiate peptides into the rat cerebral ventricle, a macrophage-like cellular response. *Brain Res. Bull.* **10**: 523.

Scholar, E. M., Rashidian, M. and Heidrick, M. L. (1980). Adenosine deaminase and purine nucleoside phosphorylase activity in spleen cells of aged mice. *Mech. Ageing Dev.* **12**: 323-329.

Schreiner, G. F., Fujiwara, K., Pollard, T. D. and Unanue, E. R. (1977). Redistribution of myosin accompanying capping of surface Ig. *J. Exp. Med.* **145**: 1393-1398.

Seshadri, R. S., Morley, A. A., Luainor, K. J. and Sorrell, J. (1979). Sensitivity of human lymphocytes to bleomycin with age. *Experientia* **35**: 233-234.

Sherr, D. H., Szewczuk, M. R. and Siskind, G. W. (1978). Ontogeny of B lymphocyte function. V. Thymic cell involvement in the functional maturation of B lymphocytes from fetal mice transferred into adult irradiated hosts. *J. Exp. Med.* **147**: 196-206.

Shipp, M. A., Stefano, G. B., D'Adamio, L., Switzer, S. N., Howard, F. D., Sinisterra, J., Scharrer, B. and Reinherz, E. (1990). Downregulation of enkephalin-mediated inflammatory responses by CD10/neutral endopeptidase 24.11. *Nature* **347**: 394-396.

Singh, J. and Singh, A. K. (1979). Age-related changes in human thymus. *Clin. Exp. Immunol.* **37**: 507-511.

Siskind, G. W., DeKruyff, R. H., Szewczuk, M., Weksler, M. E. and Goidl, E. A. (1981). Effect of age on the capacity of thymus cells to mediate B cell differentiation. In: *B Lymphocytes in the Immune Response.* Elsevier, North Holland. pp. 355-361.

Smith, E. M. and Blalock, J. E. (1981). Human lymphocyte production of corticotropin and endorphin-like substances: Association with leukocyte interferon. *Proc. Natl. Acad. Sci. USA* **78**: 7530-7535.

Smith, E. M., Morrill, A. C., Meyer, W. J. III and Blalock, J. E. (1986). Corticotropin releasing factor induction of leukocyte derived immunoreactive ACTH and endorphins. *Nature* **321**: 881-883.

Stefano, G. B. (1982). Comparative aspects of opioid–dopamine interaction. *Cell. & Mol. Neurobiol.* **2**: 167-178.

Stefano, G. B. (1988) The evolvement of signal systems: conformational matching a determining force stabilizing families of signal molecules. *Comp. Biochem. Physiol.* **90C**: 287-294.

Stefano, G. B. (1989). Role of opioid neuropeptides in immunoregulation. *Prog. in Neurobiol.* **33**: 149-159.

Stefano, G. B. (1991) Conformational matching a stabilizing signal system factor during evolution: additional evidence in comparative neuroimmunology. *Adv. Neuroimmunol.* **1**: 71-82.

Stefano, G. B., Bilfinger, T. V. and Fricchione, G. L. (1993). The immune-neuro-link and the macrophage: postcardiotomy delirium, hiv-associated dementia and psychiatry. *Prog. Neurobiol.* In press.

Stefano, G. B., Cadet, P. and Scharrer, B. (1989b). Stimulatory effects of opioid neuropeptides on locomotory activity and conformational changes in invertebrate and human immunocytes: Evidence for a subtype of delta receptor. *Proc. Natl. Acad. Sci. USA* **86**: 6307-6311.

Stefano, G. B., Kimura, T., Stefano, J. M., Finn, J., Leung, M. K., Smith, E. M. and Hughes, T. K. (1991) Age-related differences in met-enkephalin levels and numbers of opioid responsive cells in vertebrate and invertebrate immune systems. *Prog. NeuroEndocrinImmunology* **4**: 92-98.

Stefano, G. B., Leung, M. K., Zhao, X. and Scharrer, B. (1989a) Evidence for the involvement of opioid neuropeptides in the adherence and migration of immunocompetent invertebrate hemocytes. *Proc. Natl. Acad. Sci. USA* **86**: 626-630.

Stefano, G. B., Melchiorri, P., Negri, L., Hughes, T. K., and Scharrer, B. (1992). (D-Ala^2)-Deltorphin I binding and pharmacological evidence for a special subtype of delta opioid receptor on human and invertebrate immune cells. *Proc. Natl. Acad. Sci. USA* **89**: 9316-9320.

Szewczuk, M. R. and Campbell, R. J. (1980). Loss of immune competence with age may be due to auto-anti-idiotypic antibody regulation. *Nature* **286**: 164-165.

Tam, C. F. and Walford, R. L. (1978). Cyclic nucleotide levels in resting and mitogen stimulated cell suspensions from young and old mice. *Mech. Ageing Dev.* **7**: 309-320.

Tam, C. F. and Walford, R. L. (1980). Alterations in cyclic nucleotides and cyclase activities in T lymphocytes of aging humans and Down's syndrome subjects. *J. Immunol.* **125**: 1665-1670.

Thoman, M. L. and Weigle, W. O. (1981). Lymphokines and aging: Interleukin-2 production and activity in aged animals. *J. Immunol.* **127**: 2102-2106.

Thoman, M. L. and Weigle, W. O. (1982). Cell-mediated immunity in aged mice: an underlying lesion in IL 2 synthesis. *J. Immunol.* **128**: 2358-2361.

Thoman, M. L. and Weigle, W. O. (1985). Reconstitution of *in vivo* cell-mediated lympholysis responses in aged mice with Interleukin 2. *J. Immunol.* **134**: 949-952.

Thompson, J. S., Wekstein, D. R., Rhoades, J. L., Kirkpatrick, C., Brown, S. A., Roszman, T., Straus, R. and Tietz, N. (1984). The immune status of healthy centenarians. *J. Am. Geriatr. Soc.* **32**: 274-281.

Thomsen, O. and Kettel, K. (1929). Die Starke der Menschlichen Isoagglutinine und Entsperchenden Blutkorperchenrezeptoren in Verschiedenen Lebensaltern. *Z. Immunitatsforsch.* **63**: 67-93.

Utsuyama, M. and Hirokawa, K. (1987). Age-related changes of splenic T cells in mice – a flow cytometric analysis. *Mech. Ageing Dev.* **40**: 89-102.

Van Epps, D. E., Durant, D. A. and Potter, J. W. (1983a). Migration of human helper/inducor T cells in response to supernatants from Con-A-stimulated suppressor/cytotoxic T cells. *J. Immunol.* **131**: 697-703.

Van Epps, D. E., Potter, J. W. and Durant, D. A., (1983b). Production of human lymphocyte chemotactic factor by T cell subpopulations, *J. Immunol.* **130**: 2727.

Walford, D. S., Wilkens, R. F. and Decker, J. L. (1968). Impaired delayed hypersensitivity in an aging population. Association with antinuclear reactivity and rheumatoid factor. *J. Am. Med. Assn.* **203**: 832-834.

Walford, R. L. and Bergman, K. (1979). Influence of genes associated with the main histocompatibility complex on deoxyribonucleic acid excision repair capacity and bleomycin sensitivity in mouse lymphocytes. *Tissue Antigens* **14**: 336-342.

Weiner, H. L., Scribner, D. J., Schocket, A. L. and Moorhead, J. W. (1978). Increased proliferative response of human peripheral blood lymphocytes to anti-immunoglobulin antibodies in elderly people. *Clin. Immunol. Immunopath.* **9**: 356-362.

Whittingham, S., Buckley, J. D. and Mackay, I. R. (1978). Factors influencing the secondary antibody response to flagellin in man. *Clin. Exp. Immunol.* **34**: 170-178.

Woda, B. A. and Feldman, J. D. (1979). Density of surface immunoglobulin and capping on rat B lymphocytes. I. Changes with aging. *J. Exp. Med.* **149**: 416-423.

Wu, W., Pahlavani, M., Cheung, H. T. and Richardson, A. (1986). The effect of aging on the expression of Interleukin 2 messenger ribonucleic acid. *Cell. Immunol.* **100**: 224-231.

Zharhary, D. and Gershon, H. (1981). Allogeneic T cytotoxic reactivity of senescent mice: affinity for target cells and determination of cell number. *Cell. Immunol.* **60**: 470-479.

Zurawski, G., Benedik, M., Kamb, B. J., Abrams, J. S., Zurawski, S. M. and Lee, F. D. (1986). Activation of mouse T-helper cells induces abundant preproenkephalin mRNA synthesis. *Science* **232**: 772-775.

Aging and Analgesic Mechanisms

RICHARD J. BODNAR[1] and GAVRIL W. PASTERNAK[2]

[1] *Department of Psychology, Queens College, Cuny, Flushing, NY, USA*
[2] *The George C. Cotzias Laboratory of Neuro-Oncology, Memorial Sloan-Kettering Cancer Center and Department of Neurology and Neuroscience, Department of Pharmacology, Cornell University Medical College, New York, NY 10021, USA*

Introduction

The role of aging in pain perception and analgesia is a difficult area to assess. In man, it is confounded by a host of psychological factors. Many older people use pain as a means of obtaining attention while, for others, pain is a reminder of their mortality or fears, real or not, of disease. Understanding the severity of pain and its treatment requires a knowledge of the source of the pain and its meaning, as well as the background of the patient.

The evaluation of aging on the sensitivity of patients to analgesics also can be complicated by a variety of physiological factors, remote from the central systems mediating the response. For example, clinicians have long known that elderly patients are more sensitive to morphine. Although many explanations have been proposed, this increased sensitivity may be due to the accumulation of a previously unappreciated active metabolizer. In man, morphine is converted to a number of compounds, including both its 3- and 6β-glucuronides (Jaffe and Martin, 1980; McQuay and Moore, 1984; Joel *et al.*, 1986). The 3-glucuronide is inactive. Despite early studies indicating analgesic activity of morphine-6β-glucuronide (Shimomura *et al.*, 1971; Yoshimura *et al.*, 1973), most investigators did not appreciate its importance until quite recently (Osborne *et al.*, 1988; Pasternak *et al.*, 1987; Joel *et al.*, 1986). Given systemically in mice, morphine-6β-glucuronide is approximately twice as potent as morphine (Paul *et al.*, 1989). However, when administered directly into the central nervous system to bypass the blood–brain barrier, morphine-6β-glucuronide is over 100-fold more active than morphine. Morphine-6β-glucuronide is cleared renally and with chronic oral dosing its levels in blood are greater than morphine (Svensson *et al.*, 1982; Sawe *et al.*, 1983; Sawe, 1986). Normal aging is associated with a slow, progressive decline in renal function, increasing the levels of morphine-6β-glucuronide even further (Osborne *et al.*, 1986). Thus, the increased sensitivity of the elderly to morphine may be largely explained by pharmacokinetic mechanisms.

Finally, our understanding of the systems involved with pain perception and its regulation have changed drastically over the past several decades. The demonstration of electrical stimulation analgesia by Reynolds (1969) opened the possibility of discrete central mechanisms capable of pain modulation. This was followed by the demonstration of specific opioid binding sites, or receptors, within the brain (Pert and Snyder, 1973; Terenius, 1973; Simon *et al.*, 1973) which in turn led to the discovery of a large family of opioid peptides (Hughes *et al.*, 1975; Hughes, 1975; Pasternak *et al.*, 1975, 1976; Terenius and Wahlstrom, 1974). As the complexity of these systems has grown, our understanding and interpretations of earlier studies have required extensive revisions.

The purpose of these illustrations is not to suggest that it is impossible to examine the role of aging on pain perception and analgesics. Rather, we hope to point out the difficulties associated with studies in this area and the need for continued, critical review of the literature.

Role of opioid receptor multiplicity in the modulation of pain

Our understanding of various classes of opioid receptors has increased dramatically over the past two decades (Table 1). Starting with the suggestion of receptor dualism (Martin, 1967) years before the biochemical demonstration of opioid binding sites, the classification of opioid receptors has now been extended. Most investigators accept the presence of mu, kappa and delta receptors (Martin *et al.*, 1976; Lord *et al.*, 1977). Evidence from our groups and others (Wolozin and Pasternak, 1981; Pasternak and Snyder, 1975; Toll *et al.*, 1984; Goodman and Pasternak, 1985; Rothman *et al.*, 1987; Lutz *et al.*, 1984, 1985; Cruciani *et al.*, 1987; Wood *et al.*, 1982; Blurton *et al.*, 1986; for review, see Pasternak and Wood, 1986) has indicated the existence of two subtypes of mu receptors, mu_1 and mu_2, which differ in their biochemical properties, binding selectivities and, most important, their pharmacology. They were defined, in large part, by the selectivity of the antagonists naloxonazine and naloxazone for mu_1 receptors (Pasternak *et al.*, 1980a, b; Hahn *et al.*, 1982). More recently, the existence of multiple subtypes of kappa receptors has also been proposed (Martin *et al.*, 1976; Kosterlitz and Paterson, 1980; Kosterlitz *et al.*, 1981; Audiger *et al.*, 1982; Iyengar *et al.*, 1986; Wood and Iyengar, 1986; Nock *et al.*, 1988; Zukin *et al.*, 1988; Clark *et al.*, 1989; Gistrak *et al.*, 1989; Price *et al.*, 1989). The $kappa_1$ subtype has been defined by a number of investigators by its selectivity for the opioid agonist U50,488H (VonVoightlander *et al.*, 1983; Clark *et al.*, 1988) and antagonist nor-binaltorphimine (nor-BNI; Takemori *et al.*, 1988). The $kappa_2$ site was identified using binding approaches (Zukin *et al.*, 1988). Unlike the kappa receptor, it has poor affinity for U50,488H. Most recently, $kappa_3$ receptors have been reported (Price *et al.*, 1989; Clark *et al.*, 1989; Gistrak *et al.*, 1989; Paul *et al.*, 1990, 1991). These receptors, initially defined with the opiate naloxone benzoylhydrazone (NalBzoH), have the highest density within the brains of a number of species and a distinct binding selectivity. Like $kappa_2$ receptors, $kappa_3$ receptors have very poor affinity for U50,488H, as well as nor-BNI. However, $kappa_3$ are easily distinguished from the $kappa_2$ sites on the basis of the high affinity of the $kappa_3$ sites for ethylketocyclazocine and cyclazocine.

In addition to their distinct binding profiles, these sites can also be distinguished by their analgesic pharmacology (Table 2). Mu analgesia has been demonstrated both spinally and supraspinally (Paul *et al.*, 1989; Heyman *et al.*, 1988). However, the mu receptor subtypes involved in these two regions differ. β-FNA, which irreversibly blocks both mu receptor subtypes, antagonizes both supraspinal and spinal mu analgesia while naloxonazine, which is mu_1-selective, antagonizes supraspinal analgesia far more potently than spinal analgesia. Delta ligands are also potent analgesics. Although there is evidence for supraspinal mechanisms under certain conditions, spinal mechanisms are clearly far more sensitive (Porreca *et al.*, 1984). $Kappa_1$ ligands are also potent analgesics, acting predominantly at the spinal level (Takemori *et al.*, 1988). $Kappa_3$ receptor mechanisms, on the other hand, are supraspinal (Gistrak *et al.*, 1989; Paul *et al.*, 1990). $Kappa_2$ receptors have only been identified in binding studies and their pharmacology remains unknown.

Tolerance can be a problem in the use of opiates, but tolerance also provides a useful experimental approach in the investigation of these different receptor mechanisms of analgesia. Chronic administration of ligands selective for a single receptor subtype will evoke tolerance, but only to the receptor being activated. With highly selective agonists, there is virtually no cross-tolerance among the various receptor systems, providing yet another example of the independence of these analgesic systems (Gistrak *et al.*, 1989; Paul *et al.*, 1991).

Table 1. Tentative Classification of Opioid Receptor Subtypes and Opioid Binding.

	Ki (nM)						
	Mu_1	Mu_2	Delta	$Kappa_1$	$Kappa_2$	$Kappa_3$	
Mu							
Morphine	0.5 ± 0.38	2.5 ± 0.6	278 ± 49	49 ± 32		32.8 ± 2.2	
Codeine	>500	>500				>350	
DAMGO	0.5 ± 0.68	2.1 ± 0.8	>500	>350		8.2 ± 1.9	
PL-017	5.4 ± 1.6	16.5 ± 1.8	>100	>350		88.8 ± 27.8	
(-)Naloxone	1.3 ± 0.5	3.7 ± 0.7	106 ± 23	5.3 ± 1.1		8.4 ± 0.9	
(+)Naloxone	>500	>500	>500			>350	
Trimu-5	2.9 ± 0.9	14 ± 4.9	>500	>1000		314 ± 67	
Kappa							
(-)Ethylketocyclazocine	0.17 ± 0.06	0.24 ± 0.2	4.7 ± 0.5	0.21 ± 0.03	44 ± 5	1.4 ± 0.5	
(+)Ethylketocyclazocine				>350		>350	
Ketocyclazocine				1.8 ± 0.5		4.5 ± 0.8	
U50,488	370 ± 76	>500	>500	6.1 ± 1.3	484 ± 110	>350	
Nalorphine	0.8 ± 0.6	1.4 ± 0.2	32 ± 16	3.0 ± 1.6		5.4 ± 2.1	
Tifluadom				0.87 ± 0.24	39 ± 26	6.5 ± 1.2	
Mr2034				1.6 ± 0.14		2.3 ± 0.18	
Mr2266						1.0 ± 0.15	
(-)SKF10,047				2.9 ± 0.77		6.9 ± 0.97	
(+)SKF10,047				>350		>350	
WIN44,441				0.32 ± 0.12		0.2 ± 0.06	
(-)Levallorphan	0.25 ± 0.17	1.0 ± 0.2	5.4 ± 0.8	0.95 ± 0.12		2.2 ± 0.56	
(+)Levallorphan	>500	>500	>500			>350	
Levorphanol				8.1 ± 0.93		5.6 ± 1.2	
NalBzoH	0.3 ± 0.1	0.8 ± 0.2		0.60 ± 0.32		0.9 ± 0.19	
Cyclazocine				0.99 ± 0.16	65 ± 20	1.5 ± 0.59	
Pentazocine				11.8 ± 3.8		79.5 ± 16.8	
Nalbuphine				3.28 ± 1.2		5.8 ± 1.1	
nor-BNI	27.5 ± 8.9	115 ± 15	23.5 ± 5.8	3.5 ± 0.96		103 ± 8.5	
Delta							
DPDPE	82 ± 19	457 ± 149	2.9 ± 0.7	>350	>10,000	>350.	
DADL	0.9 ± 0.83	7.2 ± 3.1	1.9 ± 0.2	>350		85.9 ± 17.3	
Metkephamid	0.3 ± 0.05	0.9 ± 0.2	2.3 ± 0.2	187 ± 53		4.3 ± 0.51	
DSLET	1.4 ± 0.8	14 ± 6.5	2.3 ± 0.8			259 ± 121	
Endogenous opioid peptides							
β-Endorphin	0.98 ± 0.14	3.1 ± 0.7	2.6 ± 0.5	80 ± 20		10.7 ± 3.9	
α-Neoendorphin	5.6 ± 1.5	19 ± 7	4.2 ± 1.4			67. ± 39	
Dynorphin A(1-17)	0.69 ± 0.16	2.2 ± 0.38	8.7 ± 1.5	0.19 ± 0.08		1.7 ± 1.2	14.2 ± 7.9
Dynorphin A(1-8)	11 ± 3.5	53. ± 10.	4.1 ± 1.1	4.3 ± 1.7	115. ± 45		
Dynorphin B	6.0 ± 1.6	17. ± 4.4	6.8 ± 1.3		63. ± 17		

Values are from the literature (Clark et al., 1988; Clark et al., 1989; Zukin et al., 1988).

Table 2. Opioid Analgesia: Receptor Subtypes Involved

Anatomical location	Receptor subtype	Some typical ligands
Supraspinal		
	mu_1	morphine
	β-endorphin	
		all the synthetic enkephalins in Table 3 with the exception of DPDPE
	$kappa_3$	naloxone benzoylhydrazone nalorphine
Spinal		
	mu_2	morphine DAMGO
	$kappa_1$	U50,488 dynorphin A
	delta	enkephalin DPDPE

Opioid peptides

The enkephalins, the first opioid peptides identified, soon led to the identification of a whole family of related peptides (Table 3; for review, see Evans *et al.*, 1988). These peptides range in size from the enkephalins, which are only five amino acids, to β-endorphin, which is comprised of 31 amino acids. They all share the same initial four amino acids (Tyr-Gly-Gly-Phe) followed by either methionine or leucine. Despite this remarkable similarity in structure, each is encoded by a discrete gene (Mains *et al.*, 1977; Roberts and Herbert, 1977; Kimura *et al.*, 1980; Noda *et al.*, 1982). Both [Met^5]enkephalin and [Leu^5]enkephalin are obtained from a larger precursor protein coded by the Proenkephalin A gene, while the dynorphins and α-neoendorphin are derived from a different precursor peptide coded by the Proenkephalin B gene. Perhaps the most interesting gene is that responsible for β-endorphin. This gene encodes proopiomelanocortin, which gives rise to adrenocorticotropic hormone (ACTH), β-endorphin, α-melanocyte and γ-melanocyte stimulating hormones (α-MSH and γ-MSH), β-lipotropin and corticotropin-like intermediate lobe peptide (CLIP). However, not all the peptides are found in all tissues. The peptide processing seems to be heavily dependent upon the tissue.

Table 3. Structure of Selected Endorphins and Their Analogs

Compound	Amino acid sequence
Endogenous opioid peptides	
[Leu[5]]Enkephalin	**TYR-GLY-GLY-PHE**-Leu-OH
[Met[5]]Enkephalin	**TYR-GLY-GLY-PHE**-Met-OH
β-Endorphin	**TYR-GLY-GLY-PHE**-Met-Thr-Ser-Glu-Lys-Ser-Gln-Thr-Pro-Leu-Lys-Asn-Ala-Ile-Ile-Lys-Asn-Ala-Tyr-Lys-Gly-Glu-OH
Dynorphin A	**TYR-GLY-GLY-PHE**-Leu-Arg-Arg-Ile-Arg-Pro-Lys-Trp-Asp-Asn-Gln-OH
Dynorphin B	**TYR-GLY-GLY-PHE**-Leu-Arg-Arg-Gln-Phe-Lys-Val-Val-Thr-OH
α-Neo-endorphin	**TYR-GLY-GLY-PHE**-Leu-Arg-Lys-Tyr-Pro-Lys-OH
Selected synthetic enkephalin analogs	
DAMEA	Tyr-D-Ala-Gly-Phe-Met-$CONH_2$
DADL	Tyr-D-Ala-Gly-Phe-D-Leu-OH
FK-33824	Tyr-D-Ala-Gly-Phe(N-CH_3)-Met(O)ol
Morphiceptin	Try-Pro-Phe-Pro-$CONH_2$
Metkephamid	Try-D-Ala-Gly-Phe(N-CH_3)-Met-$CONH_2$
DPDPE	Tyr-D-Pen-Gly-Phe-D-Pen
DSLET	Tyr-D-Ser-Gly-Phe-Leu-Thr-OH
DAMGO	Tyr-D-Ala-Gly-Me-Phe-Gly(ol)

Amino acid sequences of selected endogenous and synthetic opioid peptides. Exact sequences of longer natural peptides will vary with different species. Bold portions represent the four amino acids common to all opioid peptides occurring within the central nervous system. DAMGO has also been abbreviated as DAGO in the literature.

All of these opioid peptides are readily degraded by endopeptidases and aminopeptidases. To avoid these problems in the investigation of the various opioid peptides, a number of derivatives have been synthesized, particularly in the enkephalin series. Many utilize D-amino acids, such as D-alanine, at position 2 to stabilize the peptide. In addition, a wide number of other substitutions have been examined. By selectively altering different portions of the enkephalin molecule, chemists have developed highly stable compounds which are highly selective for delta or for mu receptors.

Biochemical effects of aging and endogenous opioid systems

The two most widely studied endogenous opioids in aging processes have been β-endorphin and the enkephalins. Reductions in β-endorphin levels have been observed in the hypothalamus and striatum, but not in the median eminence and frontal cortex of aged rats (Barden *et al.*, 1981; Gambert *et al.*, 1980; Dorsa *et al.*, 1984; but see Forman *et al.*, 1981). In contrast, plasma β-endorphin levels are elevated as a function of age (Forman *et al.*, 1981). Both [Met^5]enkephalin and [Leu^5]enkephalin levels are reduced in the suprachiasmatic and premammillary hypothalamic nuclei of older male rats. Age-dependent reductions are also observed for [Met^5]enkephalin in the arcuate nucleus, and for [Leu^5]enkephalin in the paraventricular and ventro-medial hypothalamic nuclei (Dupont *et al.*, 1981). In contrast, older female rats display reductions in pituitary but not hypothalamic [Met^5]enkephalin levels (Kumar *et al.*, 1980).

The decrease in pituitary enkephalins parallels decreases in other endocrine systems, including thyroid function (Klug and Adelman, 1979; Sartin *et al.*, 1977; Denckla, 1974), gonadal function (Bruni *et al.*, 1977; Shaar *et al.*, 1975), posterior pituitary function (Zbuzek and Wu, 1982; Turkington and Everitt, 1976; Watkins and Choy, 1980; Sladek *et al.*, 1981) and adreno cortical function (Tang and Phillips, 1978; Dilman and Anisimov, 1979; Roth, 1974, 1976; Gambert *et al.*, 1980; Briton *et al.*, 1975). Further, the decrease in endogenous opioids in the central nervous system appears similar to decreases in other transmitter and peptide systems, including catecholamines (Jones and Finch, 1975; Finch, 1973; Miller *et al.*, 1976; McGeer *et al.*, 1971; Reis *et al.*, 1977), substance P (Buck *et al.*, 1981; Dupont *et al.*, 1981) and acetylcholine (e.g., Meek *et al.*, 1977), and to a lesser degree, serotonin (Finch, 1973; Simpkins *et al.*, 1977) and GABA (Govani *et al.*, 1977).

Changes in opioid binding also have been reported, but the results are somewhat contradictory and difficult to interpret. Part of the problem arises from the use of radioligands which we now know are not very selective. Furthermore, many of the studies were performed before a number of the more recently described subtypes were identified. Finally, differences in binding conditions, such as the use of buffers, temperature or salts, makes comparisons among the studies difficult. In some studies, older rats showed age-related reductions in opiate receptor number (Hess *et al.*, 1981; Messing *et al.*, 1980; Piva *et al.*, 1987), with some reports documenting the changes in the frontal cortex, striatum, amygdala, hippocampus, thalamus and midbrain. Whereas male rats failed to show specific changes in affinity of opiate binding, in another study female rats failed to display high and low affinity binding using ^3H-dihydromorphine (Hess *et al.*, 1981; Jensen *et al.*, 1980). Recently we have examined the density and affinity of a number of opioid receptor subtypes in young and aged rats. In brief, we found no significant differences in the levels of mu_1, mu_2, delta, $kappa_1$ or $kappa_3$ binding sites in rats up to 24 months old (Standifer,

Paul and Pasternak, unpublished observations). Thus, the information regarding age-related changes in specific opiate receptor subtype concentration remains difficult to reconcile.

Effect of aging on nociceptive processes and antinociception

Methodological issues

A number of general problems interfere with the analysis of aging upon nociceptive processes and antinociception. First, the nociceptive measure used across studies typically is not uniform. Second, there are highly-variable definitions of aging in animal research with rodents defined as "aged", ranging from 9 to 30 months. Third, paradigms typically employ bimodal groups, that is "young" vs. "old", in assessing aging effects. Fourth, in many studies, "elimination" criteria are not employed; i.e., are the changes in the aged animal due to the aging process itself, or some specific or general disease state of dysfunction which is associated with aging? The earlier example of morphine-6β-glucuronide illustrates this latter question. These problems arose in the early analysis of changes in basal nociceptive thresholds as a function of age. Whereas some studies found that aging increased basal pain thresholds (Pare, 1969; Nicak, 1971; Hess *et al.*, 1981), others failed to observe age-related changes (Lippa *et al.*, 1980; Saunders *et al.*, 1974; Webster *et al.*, 1976; Spratto and Dorio, 1978). Increased shock thresholds, as defined by aversion, were observed in males as compared to females across age groups, with weight acting as the determining variable for the changes (Pare, 1969). In contrast, age-related reductions were observed in both sexes when the shock thresholds were defined as an orienting response (Gordon *et al.*, 1978). However, other studies failed to observe age-related changes in shock thresholds on the jump or vocalization tests (Lippa *et al.*, 1980; Saunders *et al.*, 1974) or elevations in pain thresholds to electrical or mechanical nociceptive stimuli (Nicak, 1971). Age-dependent reactivity to heat stimuli also display equivocal results. Whereas tailflick latencies fail to change across ages in rodents (Webster *et al.*, 1976; Spratto and Dorio, 1978), hot-plate latencies decrease with age (Kavaliers *et al.*, 1983; Chan and Lai, 1982; Hess *et al.*, 1981). However, older rats display longer latencies to withdraw their tails from water at 55°C (Hess *et al.*, 1981).

Therefore, proper evaluation of aging effects upon nociceptive processes should have the following characteristics: (a) sampling of different age groups to assess whether a change in either nociceptive thresholds or antinociceptive responses occurs gradually or abruptly across the aging process; (b) multiple measures of nociception to determine whether the change in responsivity was specific to a given nociceptive modality or general across modalities; and (c) establishment of criteria that will exclude animals which may have dysfunctions which might independently alter the change in responsivity.

Aging and opiate and opioid analgesia

Analgesic sensitivity to morphine in aging rodents is reportedly reduced (Chan and Lai, 1982; Kavaliers *et al.*, 1983; Webster *et al.*, 1976), reduced and increased (Spratto and Dorio, 1978) or increased (Saunders *et al.*, 1975). These studies differ in their definitions of aging, differ in the type of nociceptive test, and typically utilize a bimodal analysis. One of our laboratories (Kramer and Bodnar, 1986a) evaluated whether aging as measured in five different groups (4, 9, 14, 19 and 24 months) altered the dose–response and time–response functions of systemic morphine analgesia as measured simultaneously by the tailflick and jump tests, and correlated these effects to age-related changes in morphine hyperthermia. The tailflick response is mediated spinally with strong supraspinal influences while the jump test measures an integrated supraspinal response. Age-related changes upon morphine analgesia (1-10 mg/kg, sc) on the tailflick test displayed a biphasic pattern with the three older groups (14-24 months) showing significant decreases in morphine analgesia 30 min after injection, and significant increases in morphine analgesia 180 min after injection. These data might be explained by such pharmacokinetic factors as delayed drug absorption and clearance or even metabolism, as suggested with morphine-6β-glucuronide. In contrast, the simultaneous analysis of aging effects on morphine analgesia on the jump test revealed equivalent reductions in analgesic magnitude across the time course and across doses for the three older groups. Further, aging failed to affect morphine hyperthermia. A simple pharmacokinetic model could not explain effects upon one measure, and failure to observe these effects on others. Therefore, it is conceivable that aging might be affecting responsivity to morphine analgesia at spinal and supraspinal levels in a differential manner.

A second study (Romeno and Bodnar, 1987) evaluated whether aging produced similar dose–response and time–response reductions in analgesia following central administration of β-endorphin. This peptide was chosen because of the previously-cited age-related reductions in β-endorphin (Barden *et al.*, 1981; Gambert *et al.*, 1980). Central administration of β-endorphin (0.1-5 μg, icv) produced analgesia in the tailflick and jump tests which did not differ as a function of age in groups of 8-, 18- and 30-month-old rats. The failure of β-endorphin analgesia to alter as a function of age stands in marked contrast to the consistent age-related reductions in β-endorphin over the life span (Barden *et al.*, 1981; Barnea *et al.*, 1982; Dorsa *et al.*, 1984; Dupont *et al.*, 1981; Forman *et al.*, 1981; Gambert *et al.*, 1980; Missale *et al.*, 1983). The failure of age-related changes in β-endorphin analgesia also contrasts with the age-related decrements in morphine analgesia. The dissociation between morphine and β-endorphin analgesia has also been observed in rats neonatally treated with monosodium glutamate, a treatment which destroys the pro-opiomelanocortin -containing cells in the hypothalamus (Bodnar *et al.*, 1980a; Krieger *et al.*, 1979). Whereas this treatment reduces morphine analgesia (Badillo-Martinez *et al.*, 1984; Bodnar *et al.*, 1980a), it fails to alter β-endorphin analgesia (Bodnar *et al.*, 1985). Some workers have suggested that β-endorphin analgesia, like morphine analgesia, may be mediated through the mu receptor (Tseng, 1981; Tseng *et al.*, 1977, 1979, 1980, 1983; Wei *et al.*, 1977) and β-endorphin analgesia is sensitive to the mu_1 antagonists naloxazone and naloxonazine (Pasternak, 1981). However, many compounds can activate more than one receptor system and it is conceivable that β-endorphin at only slightly higher doses can elicit analgesia through alternative receptor systems, possibly even the epsilon receptor subtype (Goodman *et al.*, 1983; Houghten *et al.*, 1984), and that this secondary receptor subtype may not be influenced by aging. The failure of β-endorphin to display age-related changes also differs from the observation that aging increases the proportion of N-acetylated β-endorphin (Wilkinson and Dorsa, 1986), and that this latter process decreases opioid analgesic activity (Akil *et al.*, 1981; Smyth *et al.*, 1979).

Aging and opioid/nonopioid forms of environmental analgesia

Acute exposure to certain environmental stimuli produces transient analgesic responses (see review: Bodnar *et al.*, 1980b; Watkins and Mayer, 1982; Terman *et al.*, 1984). Whereas the endogenous opioid system mediates analgesia induced under certain conditions, under others the same stimuli evoke analgesia which is opioid insensitive. For instance, acute exposure to continuous cold-water swims (CCWS) produces analgesia which shows no cross-tolerance with morphine (Bodnar *et al.*, 1978a) and is insensitive to opioid receptor antagonists (Bodnar *et al.*, 1978b; Kirchgessner *et al.*, 1982). Indeed, dissociations and collateral inhibition have been observed between the analgesic responses following CCWS and morphine (Bodnar, 1986; Yoburn *et al.*, 1987; Steinman *et al.*, 1990). In contrast, acute exposure to intermittent cold-water swims produces analgesia which is significantly reduced in morphine-tolerant rats (Girardot and Holloway, 1984a) and in rats pretreated with opiate receptor antagonists (Girardot and Holloway, 1984b). Interestingly, the magnitudes of both nonopioid CCWS analgesia and opioid ICWS analgesia are reduced in aging animals. The pattern of the significant reductions in CCWS analgesia appeared to be test-specific (Kramer and Bodnar, 1986b). On the tailflick test, CCWS analgesia was intact in rats tested at 4, 9, 14 and 19 months of age, but then declined significantly in rats at 24 months of age. On the jump test, significant reductions in CCWS analgesia occurred in the 14-month, 19-month and 24-month groups, and the pattern of these reductions grew progressively larger with age. The reductions in CCWS analgesia were not due to a concomitant age-related reduction in CCWS hypothermia. Indeed, aging produced a progressive potentiation of CCWS hypothermia. Therefore, the dissociation of analgesic and hypothermia responses to CCWS with aging implies that they do not share a common mechanism. The analgesic response following ICWS is also reduced during aging. Girardot and Holloway (1985a, b, c) found that chronic exposure to ICWS produced adaptation to the analgesic response in younger rats, but not in older, rats. Moreover, younger, but not older rats displayed greater cross-tolerance between ICWS analgesia and morphine analgesia.

Parametric variation of inescapable footshock also produces opioid and nonopioid forms of analgesia (see reviews: Watkins and Mayer, 1982; Terman *et al.*, 1984). One of these paradigms dissociated the analgesia into opioid and nonopioid based upon the body region which received shock. Whereas shock administered to the forepaws produced a opioid-sensitive analgesia, shock to the hindpaws produced an opioid-insensitive analgesia (Watkins and Mayer, 1982). Hamm and Knisely (1985, 1986a) found that aging produced significant reductions in analgesia elicited by footshock delivered to either the forepaws or hindpaws. Two other forms of environmental analgesia which are mediated in part by opioids are induced by either 2-deoxy-D-glucose (2DG) glucoprivation (Bodnar *et al.*, 1978c, 1979a, b; Spiaggia *et al.*, 1979) or food deprivation (Bodnar *et al.*, 1978d; Hamm and Lyeth, 1984; McGivern *et al.*, 1979). Aging significantly reduced 2DG analgesia in a progressive manner in rats tested at 4, 9, 14, 19 and 24 months of age (Kramer *et al.*, 1985). Notably, the hyperphagic response induced by 2DG glucoprivation (Smith and Epstein, 1969) was concomitantly reduced across the aging process to the extent that the two older groups of animals actually displayed hypophagia following 2DG (Kramer *et al.*, 1985). The analgesic response following abrupt food deprivation failed to be affected by aging in rats 4, 14 and 24 months of age (Hamm and Knisely, 1986b).

Thus, such opioid-mediated forms of environmental analgesia as ICWS, 2DG and forepaw shock display age-related reductions similar to those observed for morphine analgesia. In contrast, the opioid-mediated form of analgesia induced by food deprivation is similar to β-endorphin analgesia in that is it refractory to age-related changes. Since the precise neurochemical substrates of nonopioid forms of analgesia have not been identified, it is more difficult to link the decrements in CCWS analgesia and hindpaw shock analgesia across ages to a particular loss in neurotransmitters. One possible candidate in this regard may be acetylcholine. Both CCWS analgesia and hindpaw shock analgesia are reduced by pretreatment with scopolamine, a muscarinic cholinergic antagonist (Sperber *et al.*, 1986; Watkins *et al.*, 1984). However, Knisely and Hamm (1989) recently have demonstrated that analgesia following physostigmine, an anticholinesterase, is significantly enhanced in rats of 17 and 25 months of age relative to 3-month-old rats. These apparent contradictory findings suggest an age-related decrement in the pre-synaptic release of acetylcholine by the environmental stressors, and not a loss of post-synaptic efficacy. A second candidate involved in age-related effects upon nonopioid analgesia might be vasopressin. Vasopressin produces a non-opioid form of analgesia (Berntson and Berson, 1980; Berkowitz and Sherman, 1982; Kordower and Bodnar, 1984; Kordower *et al.*, 1982) which appears to interact with CCWS analgesia which is reduced in vasopressin-deficient Brattleboro rats (Bodnar *et al.*, 1980c), and both forms of analgesia are reduced following hypothalamic paraventricular nucleus lesions (Bodnar *et al.*, 1986; Truesdell and Bodnar, 1987). As indicated previously, vasopressin shows age-dependent decrements (Zbuzek and Wu, 1982; Turkington and Everitt, 1976; Watkins and Choy, 1980; Sladek *et al.*, 1981). However, the effects of vasopressin analgesia upon aging processes has not been evaluated.

Conclusion

In conclusion, the literature has a number of examples of changes with aging in nociception and the production of analgesia both by drugs and behavioral procedures. However, these changes are complex and will continue to require frequent reevaluation as our understanding of the mechanisms involved with these actions evolves. This area is still actively being investigated and remains an important question both for the management of pain in patients and in our understanding of the functioning of the central nervous system.

References

Akil, H., Young, E. and Watson, S. J. (1981) Opiate binding properties of naturally occurring N- and C-terminus modified beta-endorphins. *Peptides* **2**: 289-292.

Audiger, Y., Attali, B., Mazsarguil, H. and Cros, J. (1982). Characterization of [^{3}H]etorphine binding in guinea pig stratium after blockade of mu and delta sites. *Life Sci.* **31**: 1287-1290.

Badillo-Martinez, D., Kirchgessner, A. L., Butler, P. D. and Bodnar, R. J. (1984). Monosodium glutamatate and morphine analgesia test-specific effects. *Neuropharmacol.* **23**: 1141-1149.

Barden, N., Dupont, A., Labrie, F., Merand, Y., Rouleau, D. and Vaudry, H. (1981). Age-dependent changes in the beta-endorphin content of discrete rat brain nuclei. *Brain Res.* **208**: 209-212.

Berkowitz, B. Z. and Sherman, S. (1982). Characterization of vasopressin analgesia. *J. Pharmacol. Exp. Ther.* **220**: 329-334.

Berntson, G. G. and Berson, B. S. (1980). Antinociceptive effects of intraventricular or systemic administration of vasopressin in the rat. *Life Sci.* **26**: 455-459.

Blurton, P. A., Broadhurst, A. M., Wood, M. D. and Wyllie, M. G. (1986). Is there a common, high-affinity opioid binding site in rat brain? *J. Receptor Res.* **6**: 85-93.

Bodnar, R. J. (1986). Neuropharmacological and neuroendocrine substrates of stress-induced analgesia. *Ann. N.Y. Acad. Sci.* **467**: 345-360.

Bodnar, R. J., Abrams, G. W., Zimmerman, E. A., Krieger, D. T., Nicholson, G. and Kizer, J. S. (1980a). Neonatal monosodium glutamate: effects upon analgesic responsivity and immunocytochemical ACTH/beta-lipotropin. *Neuroend.* **30**: 280-284.

Bodnar, R. J., Kelly, D. D., Brutus, M. and Glusman, M. (1980b). Stress-induced analgesia: neural and hormonal determinants. *Neurosci. Biobehav. Rev.* **4**: 87-100

Bodnar, R. J., Kelly, D. D., Brutus, M., Mansour, A. and Glusman, M. (1979b). Differential effects to hypophysectomy upon analgesia induced by two glucoprivic stressors and morphine. *Pharmacol. Biochem. Behav.* **11**: 303-308.

Bodnar, R. J., Kelly, D. D., Spiaggia, A. and Glusman, M. (1978d). Biphasic alterations of nociceptive thresholds induced by food deprivation. *Physiol. Psychol.* **6**: 391-395.

Bodnar, R. J., Kelly, D. D., Spiaggia, A., Ehrenberg, C. and Glusman, M. (1978b). Dose-dependent reductions by naloxone of analgesia induced by cold-water stress. *Pharmacol. Biochem. Behav.* **8**: 667-672.

Bodnar, R. J., Kelly, D. D., Steiner, S. S. and Glusman, M. (1978a). Stress-produced analgesia and morphine-produced analgesia: lack of cross-tolerance. *Pharmacol. Biochem. Behav.* **8**: 661-666.

Bodnar, R. J., Portzline, T. and Nilaver, G. (1985). Differential alterations in opioid analgesia following neonatal monosodium glutamate treatment. *Brain Res. Bull.* **15**: 299-305.

Bodnar, R. J., Truesdell, L. S., Haldar, J., Aral, I. A., Kordower, J. H and Nilaver, G. (1986). Elimination of vasopressin analgesia following lesions placed in the rat hypothalamic paraventricular nucleus. *Peptides* **7**: 111-117.

Bodnar, R. J., Kelly, D. D., Brutus, M., Mansour, A. and Glusman, M. (1978c). 2-deoxy-D-glucose-induced decrements in operant and reflex pain thresholds. *Pharmacol. Biochem. Behav.* **9**: 543-549.

Bodnar, R. J., Kelly, D. D., and Glusman, M. (1979a). 2-deoxy-D-glucose analgesia: influence of opiate and monopiate factors. *Pharmacol. Biochem. Behav.* **11**: 297-301.

Bodnar, R. J., Zimmerman, E. A., Nilaver, G. F., Mansour, A., Thomas, L. W., Kelly, D. D. and Glusman, M. (1980c). Dissociation of cold-water swim and morphine analgesia in Brattleboro rats with diabetes insipidus. *Life Sci.* **26**: 1581-1590.

Briton, G. W., Rotenberg, S. and Adelman, R. (1975). Impaired regulation of corticosterone levels during fasting in aged rats. *Biochem. Biophys. Res. Comm.* **64**: 184-188.

Bruni, J. F., Huang, H. H., Marshall, S. and Meites, J. (1977). Effects of single and multiple injections of synthetic GnRH on serum LH, FSH and testosterone in young and old male rats. *Biol. Reprod.* **17**: 309-321.

Buck, S. H., Deshmukh, P. P., Burks, T. F. and Yamamura, H. I. (1981). A survey of substance P, somatostatin and neurotensin levels in aging in the rat and human central nervous system. *Neurobiol. Aging* **2**: 257-264.

Chan, S. H. H. and Lai, Y. Y. (1982). Effects of aging on pain responses and analgesic efficacy of morphine and clonidine in rats. *Exp. Neurol.* **75**: 112-119.

Choukyniska, R. and Bassileva-Popova, J. G. (1977). Effect of age on the binding of ^{3}H testosterone with receptor protein from rat brain and testes. *C.R. Bulg. Sci.* **30**: 133-135.

Clark, J. A., Houghten, R. and Pasternak, G. W. (1988). Opiate binding in calf thalamic membranes: a selective mu_1 binding assay. *Mol. Pharmacol.* **34**: 308-317.

Clark, J. A., Liu, L., Price, M., Hersh, B., Edelson, M., and Pasternak, G. W. (1989). Kappa opiate receptor multiplicity: Evidence for two U50,488-sensitive k_1 subtypes and a novel k_3 subtype. *J. Pharmacol. Exp. Ther.* **251**: 461-468.

Cruciani, R. N., Lutz, R. A., Munson, P. J. and Rodbard, D. (1987). Naloxonazine effects on the interaction of enkephalin analogs with mu-1, mu and delta opioid binding sites in rat brain membranes. *J. Pharmacol. Exp. Ther.* **242**: 15-20.

Denckla, W. D. (1974). Role of the pituitary and thyroid glands in the decline of minimal O_2 consumption with age. *J. Clin. Invest.* **53**: 572-581.

Dilman, V. M. and Anisimov, V. N. (1979). Hypothalamic mechanisms of aging and of specific age pathology. I. Sensitivity threshold of hypothalamo-pituitary complex to homeostatic stimuli in the reproductive system. *Exp. Gerontol.* **14**: 161-174.

Dorsa, D. M., Smith, E. R. and Davidson, J. M. (1984). Immunoreactive beta-endorphin and LHRH levels in the brains of aged male rats with impaired sex behavior. *Neurobiol. Aging* **5**: 115-120.

Dupont, A., Savard, P., Merand, Y., Labrie, F. and Boissier, J. R. (1981). Substance P. *Life Sci.* **29**: 2317-2322.

Evans, C. J., Hammond, D. L. and Frederickson, R. C. A. (1988). The opioid peptides. In: *The Opiate Receptors*, ed. G. W. Pasternak, Humana Press, Clifton, NJ, pp. 23-74.

Finch, C. E. (1973). Catecholamine metabolism in the brain of aging male mice. *Brain Res.* **52**: 261-276.

Forman, L. J., Sonntag, W. E., VanVugt, D. A. and Meites, J. (1981). Immunoreactive beta-endorphin in the plasma, pituitary and hypothalamus of young and old male rats. *Neurobiol. Aging* **2**: 281-284.

Gambert, S. R., Garthwiate, T. L., Pontzer, C. H. and Hagen, T. C. (1980). Age-related changes in central nervous system beta-endorphin and ACTH. *Neuroend.* **31**: 252-255.

Girardot, M.-N. and Holloway, F. A. (1984a). Intermittent cold-water swim analgesia in rats: cross tolerance to morphine. *Pharmacol. Biochem. Behav.* **20**: 631-633.

Girardot, M.-N. and Holloway, F.A. (1985a). Effect of age and long-term stress experience on adaptation to stress analgesia in mature rats: role of opioids. *Behav. Neurosci.* **99**: 411-422.

Girardot, M.-N. and Holloway, F.A. (1985b). Naltrexone antagonizes the biobehavioral adaptation to cold-water stress in rats. *Pharmacol. Biochem. Behav.* **22**: 769-779.

Girardot, M.-N. and Holloway, F.A. (1985c). Chronic stress, aging and morphine analgesia: chronic stress affects the reactivity to morphine in young mature but not old rats. *J. Pharmacol. Exp. Ther.* **233**: 545-553.

Girardot, M.-N. and Holloway, F.A. (1984b). Cold-water stress in rats: differential effects of naltrexone. *Physiol. Behav.* **32**: 547-555.

Gistrak, M. D., Paul, D., Hahn, E. F. and Pasternak, G. W. (1989). Pharmacological actions of a novel mixed opiate agonist/antagonist: naloxone benzoylhydrazone. *J. Pharmacol. Exp. Ther.* **251**: 469-476.

Goodman, R. N., Houghten, R. A. and Pasternak, G. W. (1983). Autoradiography of ^{3}H-beta-endorphin binding in brain. *Brain Res.* **288**: 334-337.

Goodman, R. R. and Pasternak, G. W. (1985). Visualization of mu_1 opiate receptors in rat brain using a computerized autoradiographic subtraction technique. *Proc. Nat. Acad. Sci. U.S.A.* **82**: 6667-6671.

Gordon, W. C., Scobie, S. R. and Frankel, S. E. (1978). Age-related Sprague-Dawley albino rats. *Exp. Aging Res.* **4**: 23-35.

Govani, S., Loddo, P., Spano, P. F. and Trabuchi, M. (1977). Dopamine receptor sensitivity in the brain and retina of rats during aging. *Brain Res.* **138**: 565-570.

Hahn, E. F., Carroll-Buatti, M. and Pasternak, G. W. (1982). Irreversible opiate agonists & antagonists: the 14-hydroxydihydromorphinone azines. *J. Neurosci.* **2**: 572-576.

Hamm, R. J. and Knisely, J. S. (1985). Environmentally-induced analgesia: an age-related decline in an endogenous opioid system. *J. Gerontol.* **40**: 268-274.

Hamm, R. J. and Knisely, J. S. (1986a). Environmentally-induced nonopioid system. *Psychol. Aging* **1**: 195-201.

Hamm, R. J. and Knisely, J. S. (1986b). The analgesia produced by food deprivation in 4-month, 14-month and 24-month-old rats. *Life Sci.* 1509-1515.

Hamm, R. J. and Lyeth, B. G. (1984). Nociceptive thresholds following food restriction and return to free feeding. *Physiol. Behav.* **33**: 499-501.

Hess, G. D., Joseph, J. A. and Roth, G. S. (1981). Effect of age on sensitivity to pain and brain opiate receptors. *Neurobiol. Aging* **2**: 49-55.

Heyman, J. S., Williams, C. L., Burks, T. F., Mosberg, H. I. and Porreca, F. (1988). Dissociation of opioid antinociception and central gastrointestinal propulsion in the mouse: Studies with naloxonazine. *J. Pharmacol. Exper. Ther.* **245**: 238-243.

Houghten, R. A., Johnson, N. and Pasternak, G. W. (1984). ^{3}H-beta-endorphin binding in rat brain. *J. Neurosci.* **4**: 2460-2465.

Hughes, J. T. (1975). Isolation of an endogenous compound from the brain with pharmacological properties similar to morphine. *Brain Res.* **88**: 295-308.

Hughes, J., Smith, T. W., Kosterlitz, H. W., Fothergill, L. A., Morgan, B. A. and Morris, H. R. (1975). Identification of two related pentapeptides from the brain with potent opiate agonist activity. *Nature* **258**: 577-579.

Iyengar, S., Kim, H. S. and Wood, P. L. (1986). Effects of kappa opiate agonists on neurochemical and neuroendocrine indices: evidence for kappa receptor subtypes. *Life Sci.* **39**: 637-644.

Jaffe, J. H. and Martin, W. R. (1980). Opioid analgesics and antagonists. In: *Goodman and Gilman's The Pharmacological Basis of Therapeutics, 6th ed.*, eds., A. G. Gilman, L. S. Goodman and A. Gilman, Macmillan, New York, pp. 494-534.

Jensen, R. N., Martinex, J. L., McGaugh, J. L., Messing, R. B. and Vasquez, B. J. (1980). Psychobiology of aging. In: *The Aging Nervous System*, eds., G. J. Maletta and F. J. Pirozzolio, Praeger, New York.

Joel, S. P., Osborne, R. N., Nixon, N. S. and Slevin, M. L. (1986). Morphine-6-glucuronide, an important metabolite. *Lancet* **i**: 1099-1011.

Jones, V. and Finch, C. E. (1975). Aging and dopamine uptake by subcellular fractions of the C57BL/J male mouse brain. *Brain Res.* **91**: 197-215.

Kavaliers, M., Hirst, M. and Teskey, G. C. (1983). Aging, opioid analgesia and the pineal gland. *Life Sci.* **32**: 2279-2287.

Kimura, S., Lewis, R. V., Stern, A. S., Rossier, J., Stein, S. and Udenfriend, S. (1980). Probable precursors of [Leu] and [Met] enkephalin in adrenal medulla: peptides of 3-5 kilodaltons. *Proc. Natl. Acad. Sci., U.S.A.* **77**: 1681-1685.

Kirchgessner, A. L., Bodnar, R. J. and Pasternak, G. W. (1982). Naloxazone and pain-inhibitory systems: evidence for a collateral inhibition hypothesis. *Pharmacol. Biochem. Behav.* **17**: 1175-1179.

Klug, T. L. and Adelman, R. C. (1979). Altered hypothalamic-pituitary regulation of thyrotropin (TSH) in male rats during aging. *Endocrinol.* **104**: 1136-1142.

Knisely, J. S. and Hamm, R. N. (1989). Physostigmine-induced analgesia in young, middle-aged and senescent rats. *Exp. Aging Res.* **15**: 3-11.

Kordower, J. H. and Bodnar, R. J. (1984). Vasopressin analgesia: specificity of action and non-opioid effects. *Peptides* **5**: 747-756.

Kordower, J. H., Sikorszky, V. and Bodner, R. J. (1982). Central antinociceptive effects of lysine vasopressin ans an analogue. *Peptides* **3**: 613-617.

Kosterlitz, H. W. and Paterson, S. J. (1980). Characterization of opioid receptors in nervous tissue. *Proc. R. Soc. Lond.* **210**: 113-122.

Kosterlitz, H. W., Paterson, S. J. and Robson, L. E. (1981). Characterization of the kappa subtype of opiate receptor in the guinea pig brain. *Br. J. Pharmacol.* **68**: 333-342.

Kramer, E. and Bodnar, R. J. (1986a). Age-related decrements in morphine analgesia: a parametric analysis. *Neurobiol. Aging* **7**: 185-191.

Kramer, E. and Bodman, R. J. (1986b). Age-related decrements in the

Kramer, E., Sperber, E. S. and Bodnar, R. J. (1985). Age-related decrements in the analgesic and hyperphagic responses to 2-deoxy-D-glucose. *Physiol. Behav.* **35**: 929-934.

Krieger, D. T., Liotta, A. S., Nicholson, G. and Kizzer, J. S. (1979). Brain ACTH and endorphin reduced in rats with MSG arcuate nucleus lesion. *Nature* **278**: 562-563.

Kumar, M. S. A., Chen, C. L. and Huang, H. H. (1980). Pituitary and hypothalamic concentration of met-enkephalin in young and old rats. *Neurobiol. Aging* **1**: 153-155.

Ling, G. S. F. and Pasternak, G. W. (1983). Spinal and supraspinal opioid analgesia in the mouse: the role of subpopulations of opioid binding sites. *Brain Res.* **271**: 152-156.

Lippa, A. S., Pelham, R. W., Beer, B., Critchett, D. J., Dean, R. L. and Bartus, R. T. (1980). Brain cholinergic dysfunction and memory in aged rats. *Neurobiol. Aging* **1**: 13-19.

Lord, J., Waterfield, A., Hughes, J. and Kosterlitz, H. (1977). Endogenous opioid peptides: multiple agonists and receptors. *Nature* **267**: 495-499.

Lutz, R. A., Cruciani, R. A., Costa, T., Munson, P. J. and Rodbard, D. (1984). A very high affinity opioid binding site in rat brain: demonstration by computer modeling. *Biochem. Biophys. Res. Comm.* **122**: 265-269.

Lutz, R. A., Cruciani, R. A., Munson, P. J. and Rodbard, D. (1985). Mu_1: a very high affinity subtype of enkephalin binding sites in rat brain. *Life Sci.* **36**: 2233-2338.

Mains, R. E., Eipper, B. A. and Ling, N. (1977). Common precursor to corticotropins and endorphins. *Proc. Natl. Acad. Sci., U.S.A.* **74**: 3014-3018.

Martin, W. R. (1967). Opioid antagonists. *Pharmacol. Rev.* **19**: 463-521.

Martin, W. R., Eades, C. B., Thompson, J. A., Huppler, R. E. and Gilbert, P. E. (1976). The effects of morphine and nalorphine-like drugs in the nondependent and morphine-dependent chronic spinal dog. *J. Pharmacol. Exp. Ther.* **197**: 517-532.

McGeer, E. G., Fibiger, H. C., McGeer, P. L. and Wickson, V. (1971). Aging and brain enzymes. *Exp. Gerontol.* **32**: 129-131.

McGivern, R., Berka, C., Berntson, G. G., Walker, J. M., and Sandman, C. A. (1979). Effect of naloxone on analgesia induced by food deprivation. *Life Sci.* **25**: 885-888.

McQuay, H. and Moore, A. (1984). Metabolism of narcotics. *Brit. Med. J.* **288**: 237.

Meek, J. L., Bertilsson, L., Cheyney, D. L., Zailla, G. and Costa, E. (1977). Aging-induced changes in acetylcholine and serotonin content of discrete rat brain nuclei. *J. Gerontol.* **32**: 129-131.

Messing, R. B., Vasquez, B. J., Spiehler, V. R., Martinez, J. L., Jensen, R. A., Rigter, J. and McGaugh, J. L. (1980). Dihydromorphine binding in brain regions of young and aged rats. *Life Sci.* **26**: 921-927.

Miller, A. E., Shaar, C. and Riegle, G. (1976). Aging effects on hypothalamic dopamine and norepinephrine content in the male rat. *Exp. Aging Res.* **2**: 475-480.

Missale, C., Govani, S., Croce, L., Bosio, A., Spano, P. F. and Trabucci, M. (1983). Changes of beta-endorphin and met-enkephalin content in the hypothalamus-pituitary axis induced by aging. *J. Neurochem.* **40**: 20-24.

Moskowitz, A. S. and Goodman, R. R. (1985). Autoradiographic distribution of mu_1 and mu_2 opioid binding in the mouse central nervous system. *Brain Res.* **360**: 117-129.

Moskowitz, A. S. and Goodman, R. R. (1985). Autoradiographic analysis of mu_1, mu_2 and delta opioid binding in the central nervous system of C57BL/6BY and CXBK (opioid receptor deficient) mice. *Brain Res.* **360**: 108-116.

Nicak, A. (1971). Changes of sensitivity to pain in relation to postnatal development in rats. *Exp. Gerontol.* **6**: 111-114.

Nock, B., Rajpara, A., O'Connor, L. H. and Cicero, T. J. (1988). [^{3}H]U-69593 labels a subtype of kappa opiate receptor with characteristics different from that labeled by [^{3}H]ethylketocyclazocine. *Life Sci.* **42**: 2403-2412.

Noda, M., Furutani, Y., Takahashi, H., Toyosato, M., Hirose, T., Inayama, S., Nakanishi, S. and Numa, S. (1982a). Cloning and sequence analysis of cDNA for bovine adrenal preproenkephalin. *Nature* **297**: 431.

Osborne, R. J., Joel, S. P. and Slevin, M. L. (1986). Morphine intoxication in renal failure: the role of morphine-6-glucuronide. *Brit. Med. J.* **292**: 1548-1949.

Osborne, R. J., Joel, S. P., Trex, D. and Slevin, M. (1988). Analgesic activity of morphine-6-glucuronide. *Lancet* **i**: 828.

Pare, W. P. (1969). Age, sex and strain differences in the aversive threshold to grid shock in the rat. *J. Comp. Physiol. Psychol.* **69**.

Pasternak, G. W. and Snyder, S. H. (1975). Identification of novel high affinity opiate receptor binding in rat brain. *Nature* **253**: 563-565.

Pasternak, G. W. and Wood, P. L. (1986). Multiple mu opiate receptors. *Life Sci.* **38**: 1889-1898.

Pasternak, G. W., Bodnar, R. J., Clark, J. A. and Inturrisi, C. E. (1987). Morphine-6β-glucuronide, a potent mu agonist. *Life Sci.* **41**: 2845-2849.

Pasternak, G. W., Childers, S. R. and Snyder, S. H. (1980b). Naloxazone, a long-acting opiate antagonist: effects on analgesia in intact animals and on opiate receptor binding *in vitro*. *J. Pharmacol. Exp. Ther.* **214**: 455-462.

Pasternak, G. W., Childers, S. R. and Snyder, S. H. (1980a). Opiate analgesia: evidence for mediation by a subpopulation of opiate receptors. *Science* **208**: 514-516.

Pasternak, G. W., Goodman, R. and Snyder, S. H. (1975). An endogenous morphine like factor in mammalian brain. *Life Sci.* **16**: 1765-1769.

Pasternak, G. W., Simantov, R. and Snyder, S. H. (1976). Characterization of an endogenous morphine-like factor (enkephalin). in mammalian brain. *Mol. Pharmacol.* **12**: 504-513.

Paul, D., Bodnar, R. J., Gistrak, M. D. and Pasternak, G. W. (1989). Different mu receptor subtypes mediate spinal and supraspinal analgesia in mice. *Eur. J. Pharmacol.* **168**: 307-314.

Paul, D., Standifer, K. M., Inturrisi, C. E. and Pasternak, G. W. (1989). Pharmacological characterization of morphine-6β-glucuronide, a very potent morphine metabolite. *J. Pharmacol. Exp. Ther.* **251**: 477-483

Paul, D., Levison, J. A., Howart, D. H., Pick, C. G., Hahn, E. F. and Pasternak, G. W. (1990). Naloxone benzoylhydrazone (NalBzoH) analgesia. *J. Pharmacol. Exp. Ther.* **255**: 769-774.

Paul, D., Pick, C. G., Tive, L. A. and Pasternak, G. W. (1991). Pharmacological characterization of nalorphine, a k_3 analgesic. *J. Pharmacol. Exp. Ther.*

Pert, C. B. and Snyder, S. H. (1973). Opiate receptor: demonstration in nervous tissue. *Science* **179**: 1011-1014.

Porreca, F., Mosberg, H. I., Hurst, R., Hrubey, V. J. and Burks, T. F. (1984). Roles of mu, delta and kappa opioid receptors in spinal and supraspinal mediation of gastrointestinal transit effects and hot plate analysis in the mouse. *J. Pharmacol. Exp. Ther.* **230**: 341-348

Piva, F., Maggi, R., Limonta, P., Dondi, D. and Martini, L. (1987). Decrease of mu opioid receptors in the brain and in the hypothalamus of the aged male rat. *Life Sci.* **40**: 391-398.

Price, M., Gistrak, M. D., Itzhak, Y., Hahn, E. F. and Pasternak, G. W. (1989). Receptor binding of ^{3}H-naloxone benzoylhydrazone: A reversible *k* and slowly dissociable mu opiate. *Mol. Pharmacol.* **35**: 67-74.

Reis, D. J., Ross, R. A. and Joh, T. J. (1977). Changes in the activity and the amounts of enzymes synthesizing catecholamines and acetylcholine in brain, adrenal medulla and sympathetic ganglia of aged rat and mouse. *Brain Res.* **136**: 465-474.

Reynolds, D. V. (1969). Surgery in the rat during electrical analgesic induced by focal brain stimulation. *Science* **164**: 444-445.

Roberts, J. I. and Herbert, H. (1977). Characterization of a common precursor to corticotropin and beta-lipotropin: cell-free synthesis of the precursor and identification of corticotropin peptides in the molecule. *Proc. Natl. Acad. Sci., U.S.A.* **74**: 4826-4830.

Romero, M.-T. and Bodnar, R. J. (1987). Maintenance of beta-endorphin analgesia across age cohorts. *Neurobiol. Aging* **8**: 167-170.

Roth, G. S. (1974). Age related changes in specific glucocorticoid binding by steroid responsive tissues of rats. *Endocrinol.* **94**: 82-90.

Roth, G. S. (1976). Reduced glucocorticoid binding site concentrations in cortical neuronal perikarya from senescent rats. *Brain Res.* **107**: 345-354.

Rothman, R. B., Jacobson, A. E., Rice, K. C. and Herkenham, M. (1987). Autoradiographic evidence for two classes of mu opioid binding sites in rat brain using [^{125}I]FK33824. *Peptides* **8**: 1015-1021.

Sartin, J. L., Pritchett, J. F. and Marple, D. N. (1977). TSH, theophylline and cyclic AMP: in vitro thyroid activity in aging rats. *Mol. Cell. Endocrinol.* **9**: 215-222.

Saunders, D. R., Paolino, R. M., Bousquet, W. F. and Miya, T. S. (1974). Age-related responsiveness of the rat to drugs affecting the central nervous system. *Proc. Soc. Exp. Biol. and Med.* **147**: 593-595.

Sawe, J. (1986). Morphine and its 3- and 6β-glucuronides in plasma and urine during chronic administration in cancer patients. In: *Advances in Pain Research and Therapy, vol. 8*, eds., K. M. Foley and C. E. Inturrisi, Raven Press, New York, pp. 45-56.

Sawe, J., Svensson, J.-O. and Rane, A. (1983). Morphine metabolism in cancer patients on increasing oral doses--no evidence for autoinduction or dose-dependence. *Br. J. Clin. Pharmacol.* **16**: 85-93.

Shaar, C. J., Euker, J. S., Riegle, G. D. and Meites, J. (1975). Effects of castration and gonadal steroids on serum and prolactin in old and young rats. *J. Endocrinol.* **66**: 45-51.

Shimomura, K., Kamata, O., Ueki, S., Ida, S., Oguri, K., Yoshimura, H. and Tsukamoto, H. (1971). Analgesic effect of morphine glucuronides. *Tohoku J. Exper. Med.* **105**: 45-52.

Simon, E. J., Hiller, J. M. and Edelman, I. (1973). Stereo-specific binding of the potent narcotic analgesic ^{3}H-etorphine to rat brain homogenates. *Proc. Natl. Acad. Sci. U.S.A.* **70**: 1947-1949.

Simpkins, J. W., Mueller, G. P., Huang, H. H. and Meites, J. (1977). Evidence for depressed catecholamines and enhanced metabolism in aging female rats: possible relation to gonadotropin secretion. *Endocrinol.* **100**: 1672-1678.

Sladek, C. D., McNeil, T. H., Gregg, C. M., Blair, M. L., and Baggs, R. B. (1981). Vasopressin and renin response to dehydration in aged rats. *Neurobiol. Aging* **2**: 293-302.

Smith, G. P. and Epstein, A. N. (1969). Increased feeding in response to decreased glucose utilization in the rat and monkey. *Am. J. Physiol.* **217**: 1083-1087.

Smyth, D. G., Massey, D. E., Zakarian, S. and Finnie, M. D. A. (1979). Endorphins are stored in biologically active and inactive forms: isolation of alpha-N-acetyl peptides. *Nature* **279**: 252-254.

Sperber, E. S., Kramer, E. and Bodnar, R. J. (1986). Effects of muscarinic receptor antagonism upon two forms of stress-induced analgesia. *Pharmacol. Biochem. Behav.* **25**: 171-179.

Spiaggia, A., Bodnar, R. J., Kelly, D. D. and Glusman, M. (1979). Opiate and non-opiate mechanisms of stress-induced analgesia. *Pharmacol. Biochem. Behav.* **10**: 761-765.

Spratto, A. and Dorio, R. E. (1978). Effect of age on the acute morphine response in the rat. *Res. Comm. Chem. Pathol. Pharmacol.* **19**: 23-26.

Steinman, J. L., Faris, P. L., Mann, P. E., Olney, J. W., Komisaruk, B. R., Willis, W. D. and Bodnar, R. J. (1990). Antagonism of morphine analgesia by nonopioid cold-water swim analgesia: direct evidence for collateral inhibition. *Neurosci. Behav. Rev.* **14**: 1-7.

Svensson, J.-O., Rand, A., Sawe, J. and Sjoqvist, F. (1982). Determination of morphine, morphine-3-glucuronide and (tentatively). morphine-6β-glucuronide in plasma and urine using ion-pair high-performance liquid chromatography. *J. Chromatog.* **230**: 427-432.

Takemori, A. E., Ho, Y. H., Naeseth, J. S. and Portoghese, P. S. (1988). Nor-binaltorphimine, a highly selective *k*-opioid antagonist in analgesic and receptor binding assays. *J. Pharmacol. Exp. Ther.* **246**: 255-258.

Tang, F. and Phillips, J. G. (1978). Some age-related changes in pituitary-adrenal function in the male laboratory rat. *J. Gerontol.* **33**: 377-382.

Terenius, L. (1973). Characteristics of the "receptor" for narcotic analgesics in synaptic plasma membrane fractions from rat brain. *Acts Pharmacol. Toxicol.* **33**: 377-384.

Terenius, L. and Wahlstrom, A. (1974). Inhibitor(s) of narcotic receptor binding in brain extracts and in cerebrospinal fluids. *Acts Pharmacol. (Kbh). [Suppl. 1]* **33**: 55.

Terman, G. W., Shavit, Y., Lewis, J. W., Cannon, J. T. and Liebeskind, J. C. (1984). Intrinsic mechanisms of pain inhibition and their activation by stress. *Science* **226**: 1270-1277.

Toll, L., Keys, C., Polgar, W. and Low, G. (1984). *Neuropeptides* **5**: 205-208.

Truesdell, L. S. and Bodnar, R. J. (1987). Reduction in cold-water swim analgesia following hypothalamic paraventricular nucleus lesions. *Physiol. Behav.* **39**: 727-731.

Tseng, L. F. (1981). Comparison of analgesic and body temperature responses to intrathecal beta-endorphin and D-Ala-D-Leu-enkephalin. *Life Sci.* **29**: 1417-1424.

Tseng, L. F., Cheng, S. S. and Fujimoto, J. M. (1983). Inhibition of tail-flick and shaking responses by intrathecal and intraventricular D-Ala-D-Leu-enkephalin and beta-endorphin in anesthetized rats. *J. Pharmacol. Exp. Ther.* **224**: 51-54.

Tseng, L. F., Loh, H. H. and Li, C. H. (1977). Human beta-endorphin in anesthetized rats. *Biochem. Biophys. Res. Commun.* **74**: 390-396.

Tseng, L. F., Ostwald, T. J., Loh, H. H. and Li, C. H. (1979). Behavioral activities of opioid peptides and morphine sulfate in golden hamsters and rats. *Psychopharm. (Berl.)* **64**: 215-218.

Tseng, L. F., Wei, E. T., Loh, H. H. and Li, C. H. (1980). Beta-endorphin: central sites of analgesia, catalepsy and body temperature change in rats. *J. Pharmacol. Exp. Ther.* **214**: 328-332.

Turkington, M. R. and Everitt, A. V. (1976). The neurohypophysis and aging with special reference to the antidiuretic hormone. In: *Hypothalamus, Pituitary and Aging*, eds., A. V. Everitt and J. A. Burgess, C.C. Thomas, Springfield, IL.

Ueno, E., Liu, D. D., Ho, I. K. and Hoskins, B. (1988). Opiate receptor characteristics in brains from young, mature and aged mice. *Neurobiol. Aging* **9**: 279-283.

VonVoightlander, P. F., Lahti, R. A. and Ludens, J. H. (1983). U50,488: a selective and structurally novel non-mu (kappa) opioid agonist. *J. Pharmacol. Exp. Ther.* **224**: 7-12.

Watkins, L. R. and Mayer, D. J. (1982). The neural organization of endogenous opiate and nonopiate pain control systems. *Science* **216**: 1185-1192.

Watkins, L. R., Katayama, Y., Kinscheck, I. B., Mayer, D. J. and Hayes, R. (1984). Muscarinic cholinergic mediation of opiate and non-opiate environmentally induced analgesia. *Brain Res.* **300**: 231-242.

Watkins, W. B. and Choy, V. J. (1980). The impact of aging on neuronal morphology in the rat hypothalamo-neurohypophyseal system: an immunohistochemical study. *Peptides* **1**: 239-245.

Webster, G. W., Schuster, L. and Eleftheriou, B. E. (1976). Morphine analgesia in mice of different ages. *Exp. Aging Res.* **2**: 221-223.

Wei, E. T., Tseng, L. F., Loh, H. H. and Li, C. H. (1977). Comparison analogs. *Life Sci.* **21**: 321-328.

Wilkinson, C. W. and Dorsa, D. M. (1986). The effects of aging on molecular forms of beta- and gamma-endorphins in rat hypothalamus. *Neuroend.* **43**: 124-131.

Wolozin, B. L. and Pasternak, G. W. (1981). Classification of multiple morphine and enkephalin binding sites in the central nervous system. *Proc. Nat. Acad. Sci. U.S.A.* **78**: 6181-6185.

Wood, P. L. and Iyengar, S. (1986). Kappa isoreceptors: neuroendocrine and neurochemical evidence. *NIDA Research Monograph* **71**: 102-108.

Wood, P. L., Richard J. W. and Thakur, M. (1982). Mu opiate isoreceptors: differentiation with kappa agonists. *Life Sci.* **31**: 2313-2317.

Yoburn, B. C., Truesdell, L. S., Kest, B. and Inturrisi, C. R. (1987). Y facilitates non-opioid stress-induced analgesia. *Pharamacol. Biochem. Behav.* **27**: 525-527.

Yoshimura, H., Ida, S., Oguri, K. and Tsukamoto. (1973). Biochemical basis for analgesic activity of morphine-6β-glucuronide. I: Penetration of morphine-6-glucuronide in the brain of rats. *Biochem. Pharmacol.* **22**: 1423-1430.

Zbuzek, B. K. and Wu, W. (1982). Age related vasopressin changes in rat plasma and the hypothalamo-neurohypophyseal system. *Exp. Gerontol.* **17**: 133-138.

Zukin, R. S., Eghbali, M., Olive, D., Unterwald, E. M. and Tempel, A. (1988). Characterization and visualization of rat and guinea pig brain *k* opioid receptors: Evidence for k_1 and k_2 opioid receptors. *Proc. Nat. Acad. Sci. U.S.A.* **85**: 4061-4065.

The Pond Snail *Lymnaea Stagnalis* – an Animal Model for Aging Studies in the Central Nervous System

C. JANSE

Faculty of Biology, Free University De Boelelaan 1087, 1081 HV Amsterdam, The Netherlands

Introduction

The fundamental mechanisms which underly aging processes are still poorly understood. This is illustrated by the great number of theories to explain aging which exists at present (cf. Adelman and Roth, 1982; Cristofalo, 1988). These theories concern processes ranging from the molecular up to the organismic level. It should, however, be emphasized that aging of the organism involves a number of processes which interact with each other (Finch, 1988). This implies that aging studies at any level should take into account the biology and physiology of the organism. Because of their relative simplicity, lower animals might provide a good opportunity for such studies.

Several lower animal species are at present used in experimental studies of aging processes (cf. Mitchell and Johnson, 1984; Lints, 1985). As will be pointed out in the present chapter, among the lower animals molluscs, especially several gastropod species, provide suitable model systems for aging studies in the nervous and neuroendocrine systems. The nervous system of these animals is well known and contains neurons which are readily accessible for different techniques. Moreover, much is known on the biology and physiology of these animals. In the present chapter attention is especially focused on aging studies on the pond snail *Lymnaea stagnalis*.

General biology and life cycle of *Lymnaea*

The three largest animal groups are the arthropods, molluscs and vertebrates with 78%, 7% and 3% of the number of species, respectively. *Lymnaea* belongs to the molluscs, as indicated by the number of species one of the most successful animal groups. Within the group of the molluscs the gastropods form one of the main groups. They have adapted to the three major habitats on earth, i.e. marine, terrestrial and freshwater. Representatives can be found worldwide in such diverse habitats as the tropical seas, near the eternal snow line in Greenland, and in the deserts of Africa. Within the group of the gastropods, especially the pulmonates are known for their adaptation to different habitats (Newell, 1964; Russell-Hunter, 1964, 1983). This great adaptability may be related to the well-developed behavioural and organ systems of these animals which are controlled by adequate nervous and neuroendocrine systems.

Within the group of the gastropods, different types of reproduction occur. Animals of this group show gonochorism as well as hermaphroditism. Which sexual life style is used depends on individual mobility and density of natural populations (Calow, 1983). *Lymnaea* belongs to the pulmonate gastropods and has a hermaphroditic life style. Mature animals produce egg masses which contain 100-150 eggs.

During embryogenesis most gastropod species have larval stages which strongly differ from the adult stage. Consequently, they show metamorphosis. The larvae of most marine and some freshwater species of gastropods are free living. In metamorphosis, often special conditions (i.e. food) are required. This makes the particular species difficult to breed in the laboratory. Nevertheless, breeding methods for such species have been developed for the hermaphroditic marine gastropods *Aplysia californica* (Kriegstein *et al.*, 1974; Capo *et al.*, 1979) and *Tritonia diomedea* (Kempf and Willows, 1977). The larvae of pulmonate gastropods show metamorphosis within the egg. Young snails hatch from the egg capsules in their adult appearance. Pulmonates are, therefore, relatively easy to breed. In our laboratory the pulmonate *Lymnaea stagnalis* is cultured in a semi-automatic system with continuous water refreshment, which produces several tens of thousands of snails of different age a year (van der Steen *et al.*, 1969; Janse *et al.*, 1988).

The maximum age among molluscs differs considerably. Comfort (1957) gives a great number of data on molluscan longevity, most of it concerning animals under natural conditions. The shortest living gastropods occur among *Lymnaea* species; maximum life spans of 139 days to 3 years have been reported. The marine gastropod *Aplysia californica* has a maximum life span of about 10 months (Hirsch and Peretz, 1984). Land pulmonates belong to the longest living gastropods. Reports are known of *Helix* specimens living 15 years in breeding conditions (Comfort, 1957). In our laboratory in standard conditions the pond snail *Lymnaea* has a maximum life span of 22 months (Janse *et al.*, 1988). It goes without saying that species with a relatively short life span are most suitable for experimental aging studies.

Aging and survival of *Lymnaea*

Aging in a population is characterized by an increase of the age-specific death rate with age (Comfort, 1979). In many natural populations death rate is independent of age. In such populations the number of survivors decreases exponentially with age. Animal populations maintained in laboratory conditions often show an age-related increase in the age-specific death rate. As a consequence, the survival curves become more rectangular. Survival curves of molluscs cultured in laboratory conditions have been published only for a few species. For *Aplysia,* survival has been studied of captured animals kept under laboratory conditions. Under these conditions this species has a rectangular survival curve and an increase of the age-specific death rate with age (Hirsch and Peretz, 1984), indicating that aging occurs.

In *Lymnaea,* cultured under laboratory conditions, the age-specific death rate increases with age (Slob and Janse, 1988). In this species (Janse *et al.*, 1988; Slob and Janse, 1988) and in other pulmonates (Comfort, 1979) rectangular survival curves occur in breeding conditions (Fig. 1). In *Lymnaea,* survival curves could be fitted with the Gompertz and Weibull functions (Slob and Janse, 1988). On the basis of these survival data it has been concluded that, in breeding conditions, *Lymnaea* ages (Janse *et al.*, 1988; Slob and Janse, 1988). Mortality in *Lymnaea* increases at an age of about 8 months, the median life span is reached at about 12 months and the maximum life span at about 22 months (Fig. 1; Janse *et al.*, 1988; Slob and Janse, 1988).

In *Lymnaea,* death rate can suddenly increase, probably due to a water-transmittable disease (Janse *et al.*, 1988). This makes it necessary in aging studies to discriminate between healthy and infected populations. Such a discrimination can be made on the basis of the shape and parameters of survival curves. With maximum-likelihood methods, predictions of survival curves and their parameters can now be made on the basis of the Weibull function, even with only 25% of the death rate data (75% survival) (Slob and Janse, 1988). This makes it possible in cross-sectional aging studies to compare the quality of experimental animals from different cultures. In this way, animal cultures which are used for aging studies are now screened for abnormal death rates.

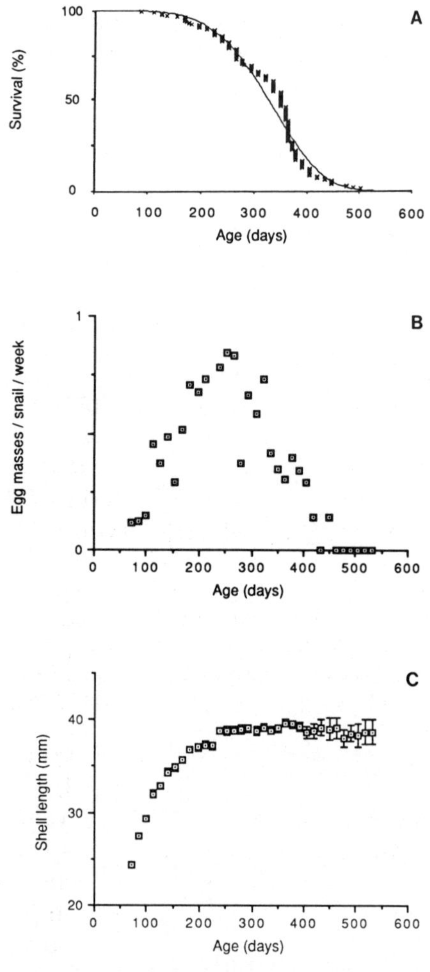

FIG. 1. Longitudinal study of a snail population of 200 snails kept under standard conditions. A. Survival; the continuous line represents the Weibull function (Slob and Janse, 1988) fitted through the survival data. The culture was terminated at an age of about 540 days; at that age 3 animals were left. The median survival age of the population was 329 ± 6 (s.e.) days. B. Mean number of egg masses produced per snail per week. Note that at the end of the culture period 5 animals did not lay eggs for about 100 days. C. Growth in the population as indicated by mean shell length (and s.e.). x: occurrences of individual dead animals (From Janse *et al.*, 1989).

According to Kirkwood (1985), animals keep a balance between energy investments in maintenance, growth and repair on the one hand and reproductive activity on the other hand. This implies that changes in for example, reproductive activity or growth will have consequences for other types of physiological activities of the organism. It is therefore of importance in aging studies to know if and how energy-consuming processes like growth and reproduction change with age.

Molluscs like other animal species show a von Bertalanffy type of growth; after a period of rapid growth, growth rate decreases (Kooijman, 1988). *Lymnaea* ceases growth at an age of about 8 months. Figure 1 shows that this is about the same age at which reproduction starts to decrease. In culture conditions, *Lymnaea* reaches a shell length of about 4 cm (Janse *et al.*, 1988; 1989).

Of only a few molluscan species is the fate of the animals after their reproductive period known. The opistobranch *Aplysia* (Van Heukelem, 1979) and the cephalopod *Octopus* die shortly after cessation of reproductive activity. In *Octopus*, this is caused by inhibition of eating behaviour after the production of eggs (Wodinsky, 1977). Only in pulmonate snails has a distinct postreproductive period been described (Comfort, 1979). The postreproductive period starts after growth has ceased (Comfort, 1957, 1979). In cultured *Lymnaea*, female reproductive activity increases up to an age of about 8 months; thereafter, it decreases with age (Fig. 1). As described above, at about this age death rate of *Lymnaea* increases notably in our cultures.

In *Lymnaea*, food consumption affects reproductive activity and growth (Scheerboom, 1978; Dogterom *et al.*, 1984). Recent experiments showed that food consumption also affects survival of *Lymnaea*. Figure 2 demonstrates this for three groups of animals hatched at the same time but kept under different feeding conditions. The groups were kept in the same breeding tank in separate compartments. Because animals of these groups were also used for physiological experiments, the cultures were terminated before 0% survival was reached (see also Janse *et al.*, 1991). On the basis of the survival data the survival curves of the different populations could be estimated with the Weibull function (Slob and Janse, 1988). Figure 2 shows that the culture fed once a week had a longer life expectancy than those fed *ad libitum* and once every two weeks, respectively. The figure also shows that reproductive activity in the groups differed considerably. The *ad libitum* fed animals had a very high reproductive rate, whereas the two other groups had a very low rate of reproduction. Animals fed at a rate of once every two weeks were probably underfed; this group lived much shorter than the two other groups.

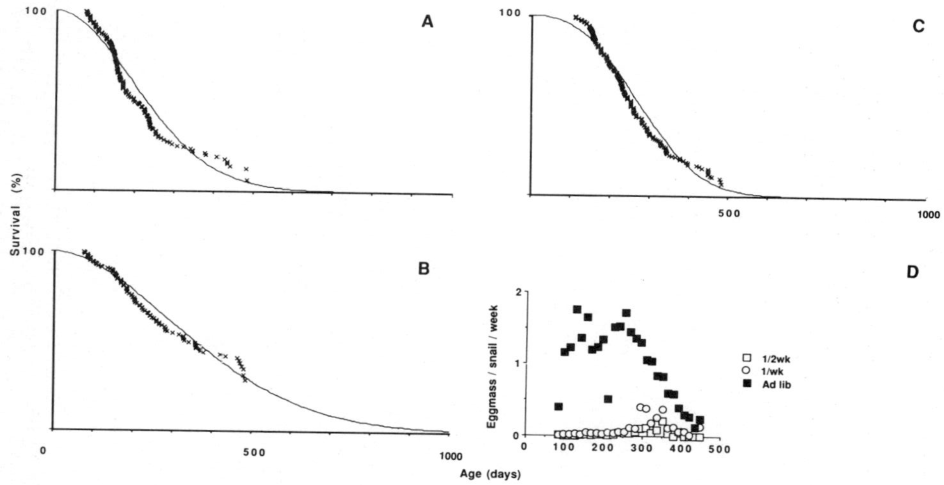

FIG. 2. A - C. Survival percentages of *Lymnaea* as plotted against age at different feeding conditions. At the start of the experiment groups consisted of 200 animals aged 40 days. The survival percentages have been corrected for the numbers of animals sampled for electrophysiological measurements. Each individual that died is indicated by x. The continuous lines represent the survival curves as calculated according to the Weibull model (cf. Slob and Janse, 1988). From the Weibull model it was calculated that the median age in A (fed lettuce once every 2 weeks) was 225 ± 10 (s.e.) days, in B (fed once a week) 355 ± 20 days and in C (fed *ad libitum*) 275 ± 9 days. Animals in group A probably represent malnutritive animals. D. Egg-laying frequency of *Lymnaea* at different feeding conditions. The cultures are the same as those in A - C. Egg-laying was calculated at two-week intervals by dividing the number of egg masses by the number of animals alive (From Janse *et al.*, 1991).

In mammals, food restriction increases life span (Weindruch and Walford, 1988) and diminishes the age-related decrease of nervous functions (Levin *et al.*, 1981; Massoro, 1988). The mechanisms along which feeding conditions affect survival are, however, still unknown. Indications exist that glucose levels in the blood are of importance (Massoro *et al.*, 1989). In *Lymnaea,* it is known that feeding affects glucose levels in the blood (Scheerboom, 1978) and that these levels are part of hormonal control systems (Joosse, 1988).

The nervous and neuroendocrine systems of *Lymnaea*

Molluscan and vertebrate neurons share a common plan, and their biophysical, biochemical and integrative properties are basically the same (Kandel, 1976). This implies that at the neuronal level vertebrate and molluscan nervous systems are functionally similar. They differ, however, in the degree of organization. The organization of vertebrate nervous systems is more complicated than that of molluscs.

Lymnaea has a nervous system which is typical for molluscs. In molluscs, the CNS consists of a number of ganglia connected by connectives (between different ganglia) and commissures (between paired ganglia). In gastropods, the ganglia are clearly separated. In addition to the CNS, molluscs have a peripheral nervous system which is able to mediate reflex behaviour (Janse, 1974; Mpitsos and Lukowiak, 1985). Molluscan neurons are essentially monopolar; in this aspect they resemble the vertebrate sensory neuron. In the CNS, their cell bodies are situated in the periphery of the ganglion and they send their axons to the central region of the ganglion, the neuropil. In the neuropil, they make synaptic contacts with axons originating from neurons in the same ganglion or in other ganglia, or with axons from peripheral neurons. Chemical and electrical synapses occur. Clusters of synapses can be found on the axon hillock and/or on the branching axon. Axo-somatic synaptic contacts occur as well (Roubos, 1984).

The CNS of many molluscs contains giant neurons situated underneath the perineurium. These properties make these neurons relatively easily accessible for different techniques, thus permitting the combination of physiological, biochemical, morphological and molecular studies. Therefore, this CNS is an ideal model system for the study of fundamental mechanisms of the nervous sysem. At present, especially gastropod nervous systems are popular for studies of fundamental mechanisms underlying behaviour. In these animals the diameter of the nerve cell bodies may even exceed 1 mm. Individual neurons can be identified by their position, shape, and electrical characteristics. Moreover, in gastropods such as *Lymnaea* the neurons are differently coloured, which makes them easy to identify visually.

This makes it possible in these animals to relate activities of individual nerve cells to specific behaviours. Among the molluscs, especially in *Lymnaea* and *Aplysia*, the behavioural function of a great number of identified nerve cells is now known (Kandel, 1976, 1979; Benjamin, 1983; Winlow and Haydon, 1985; Geraerts *et al.*, 1988; van der Wilt *et al.*, 1987, 1988).

In molluscs an intimate relationship exists between the nervous and the neuroendocrine system, since the majority of the neuroendocrine (neurosecretory) cells are incorporated in the CNS. In addition, like in other animals, neurosecretory and "common" neurons resemble each other in many aspects. They have similar integrative and electrical properties and in principle similar mechanisms to release their products (cf. Joosse *et al.*, 1982; Joosse, 1986). Neurosecretory cells occur in groups or dispersed in the CNS and produce neurohormones. These neurons have release areas located underneath the perineurium of ganglia, connectives, commissures and peripheral nerves (Wendelaar Bonga, 1970; Joosse, 1979). Contrary to vertebrates, molluscs only possess a few (1-3) endocrine organs. Consequently nearly all neurohormones in molluscs act directly on non-endocrine targets. In the pond snail *Lymnaea stagnalis* only one endocrine organ is known, the paired dorsal bodies (DBs). The DBs are located on the cerebral ganglia, and control oocyte growth and maturation and secretory activity of the female accessory sex organs (Geraerts and Joosse, 1975). Like in vertebrates, neurohormones in molluscs control physiological processes such as growth, reproduction, ionic and energy metabolism, blood volume and heart rate. In addition, group specific functions such as shell growth are under hormonal control (for reviews see Joosse and Geraerts, 1983; Joosse, 1988).

In the last decade in studies on the nervous system much attention has been paid to peptides. Moreover, there is an increasing interest for the role of peptides in aging of the nervous system (Janse *et al.*, 1991a). Neuropeptides occur in molluscs in a great molecular diversity (up to 100 in one species: cf. Joosse, 1986). Immunocytochemical studies have shown that a great number of these peptides are vertebrate-like. On the other hand, peptides related to those first described in molluscs have been found in the vertebrate brain (Boer and van Minnen, 1988). Evidence is accumulating rapidly that neuropeptides function both at synaptic sites as well as in more diffuse ways of transmission in molluscs and vertebrates (Joosse, 1986).

In molluscs, neuropeptides play a role in many functions including neuroendocrine control systems (Joosse, 1986), modulation of neuronal networks underlying behaviour (Murphy *et al.*, 1985; van der Wilt *et al.*, 1988), induction of complex behaviours such as egg laying (Geraerts *et al.*, 1988), synaptic control of muscles (Cottrell *et al.*, 1983; Schot *et al.*, 1983; Whim and Lloyd, 1990) or neurons (Boer *et al.*, 1984) and neurite outgrowth and synapse formation (Bulloch, 1987). Coexistence of several peptides in one neuron has been shown in *Lymnaea* in many neurons including the caudo dorsal cells (CDCs) and in *Aplysia* in the bag cells (Geraerts *et al.*, 1983, 1988; Scheller *et al.*, 1983). These multiple peptides function probably in the control of different aspects of egg-laying behaviour of the respective snails (Geraerts *et al.*, 1988). Peptidergic neurons involved in modulation or induction of behaviour often seem to be multifunctional.

Especially in gastropods, pharmacological studies have produced evidence of many substances being putative transmitters. ACh is at present the only transmitter substance which can fulfil all the requirements for being a neurotransmitter. In addition to ACh, noradrenaline, dopamine, 5-hydroxytryptamine, histamine, GABA and several amino acids are likely neurotransmitters in molluscs. These substances are present in the nervous system and responses of central neurons to these substances have been studied extensively (for a review see Rózsa, 1984). Indications of coexistence of different classical transmitters in one neuron have been obtained in *Helix* by Cottrell (1977).

Age-related changes in the nervous and neuroendocrine systems of *Lymnaea*

Changes in the neuroendocrine system involved in reproductive control

In *Lymnaea*, egg laying is controlled by hormones secreted by the DBs (DB-hormone) and the CDCs (CDC-hormone). DB-hormone controls cellular differentiation, growth and synthetic activity of the accessory sex organs. CDC-hormone controls ovulation, egg-laying behaviour and synthesis and packaging of the eggs (Joosse, 1988). Just before the start of ovulation and egg laying the CDCs become electrically active. Upon activation, they secrete CDC-hormone and multiple other peptides in the haemolymph which induce a stereotyped pattern of overt and covert behaviours which terminates in the deposition of an egg mass (Fig. 3) (see also Geraerts *et al.*, 1988).

Longitudinal studies showed that egg-laying activity changes with age (Fig. 1). In young animals, egg-laying activity initially increases with age. Up to an age of about 250 days, the number of egg masses produced per snail and the number of eggs per egg mass increases with age. This has been ascribed to developmental processes (Geraerts and Joosse, 1975; Bohlken and Joosse, 1982; Janse *et al.*, 1989). At an age of about 250 days egg laying starts to decrease again and egg mass and egg production decreases (Janse *et al.*, 1989). At an age of about 500 days most animals have ceased egg-laying activity and are in their postreproductive period (Fig. 1).

Cross-sectional studies (Janse *et al.*, 1989) showed that the increase in reproduction holds for the frequency of oviposition as well as for the percentage of animals that shows egg-laying activity. The decline in egg-laying activity appeared also to be composed of a decrease of the egg-laying frequency of individual animals and of a simultaneously occurring decrease of the percentage of animals that lay eggs. From these studies it also appeared that there is a considerable individual variability in the age at which *Lymnaea* reaches full maturity and lay eggs and in the age at which this species enters its postreproductive state, respectively.

Upon injection of synthetic CDC-hormone, old *Lymnaea* that had ceased female reproductive activity could still lay eggs (Janse *et al.*, 1990). Obviously, the peripheral sex organs are still intact and reproductive cessation is in these animals due to changes in central mechanisms controlling reproduction. The injection experiments also showed that old animals that had ceased reproduction responded less to CDC-hormone injection than old still reproductive animals of the same age. No differences in CDC-hormone responsiveness were found between old and young reproductive animals. This indicates that differences in sensitivity of the female sex organs to CDC-hormone are not related to differences in age but to differences in sexual activity.

It has been suggested that in *Lymnaea* sensitivity of female reproductive organs to CDC-hormone is controlled by hormone secreted by the DBs (Dogterom *et al.*, 1983, 1984; Joosse, 1988). In this view it is conceivable that in some old animals DB-hormone levels in the blood decrease due to deterioration of the DBs. These low DB-hormone levels may result in a decrease in sensitivity of peripheral female reproductive organs to CDC-hormone. Degeneration of DBs in old animals has indeed been reported (Joosse, 1964). Implantation of cerebral ganglia, including the DBs of young animals (3 months of age) into old animals (10 months) at which egg laying was reduced, increased the egg-laying frequency. Implantation of cerebral ganglia with DBs of old animals into old animals did not affect egg-laying frequency (Janse *et al.*, 1991b). This indeed indicates that changes in a humoral factor are involved in the age-related decrease of female reproduction.

Injection of homogenates of CDCs of old animals that ceased egg laying into young reproductive animals produced ovulation in the injected animals. This indicates that the CDCs of old non-reproductive animals still contain active CDC-hormone (Janse *et al.*, 1990). Obviously old non-reproducing animals do not release CDC-hormone (in sufficient amounts).

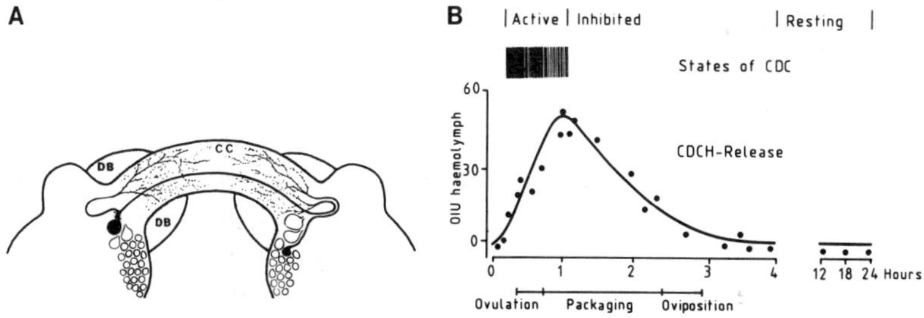

FIG. 3. A. Ventral view of the cerebral ganglia of *Lymnaea* with the morphology of the CDCs. The branching pattern of two different types of CDC is indicated, one with an axon at the ipsilateral side only and one with the second axon crossing to the contralateral side. Electrical activity in the clusters of CDCs results in release of CDC-hormone and other peptides at the periphery of the commissure. B. Diagram of interrelations of electrical activity of CDCs, release of CDC-hormone and overt and covert behaviours induced by an egg-laying stimulus (water change). DB: dorsal body; CC: cerebral commissure; OIU: Ovulation Inducing Units as measured by bioassay (Geraerts *et al.*, 1984) (From Janse and Joosse, 1989).

It is known that changes in excitability of the CDCs underly the egg-laying cycle of young *Lymnaea* (Fig. 3) (see also Kits, 1980). Preceding oviposition, the CDCs are electrically active and in the active state (Ter Maat *et al.*, 1986). Immediately after oviposition they are in a refractory (inhibited) state which gradually changes into the resting state in which the CDCs can be brought into afterdischarge (Kits, 1980). In addition to the cyclic changes in excitability, the CDCs are also influenced by external and internal conditions (Ter Maat *et al.*, 1982, 1983).

Electrophysiological experiments showed that CDCs of old non-reproducing animals can still generate an afterdischarge upon electrical stimulation. This indicates that in these animals the CDCs are in the resting state (Janse *et al.*, 1990). It is therefore concluded that cessation of female reproductive activity is not primarily due to the CDCs not being able to produce a discharge. These results do not exclude the possibility that in postreproductive animals the CDCs are periodically electrically active and, although they contain effective CDC-hormone, they do not release the hormone into the blood.

Preliminary EM observations, however, revealed that CDCs of postreproductive animals brought into afterdischarge by electrical intracellular stimulation still showed morphological characteristics of active secretion (E. W. Roubos, personal communication; see also Roubos and van der Wal-Divendal, 1980). This may indicate that CDCs in old non-reproducing animals can still release CDC-hormone but probably do not do so because they remain electrically silent.

Electrophysiological studies (Janse *et al.*, 1990) also showed that the CDCs of old postreproductive animals have a much longer lasting discharge upon electrical stimulation than those of both old and young reproductive animals. This difference might be related to the cessation of CDC activity in postreproductive animals. For, after spontaneous CDC activity has ceased the CDCs will no longer show the discharge-induced pulsatory release of their peptides. This may imply that the peptides in the CDCs of these animals accumulate as the animal continues to age. These peptides include peptides with autotransmitter function which are of importance for simultaneous activation of the CDCs (Ter Maat *et al.*, 1982). It is conceivable that during CDC activity, due to this accumulation, peptides with autotransmitter function are secreted over a longer period and that this results in a longer lasting afterdischarge. An increased secretion of autotransmitter may also explain the high amplitude of the depolarizing afterpotential, which is thought to be the result of chemical communication between the CDCs (Ter Maat *et al.*, 1988) in old non-laying snails (Janse *et al.*, 1990). In this view the electrophysiological differences between CDCs of reproductive and postreproductive animals are not a direct consequence of aging but a secondary result of lack of activation of the CDCs.

Egg-laying inducing stimuli such as the clean water stimulus do not induce egg laying in old animals that had ceased female reproductive activity (Janse *et al.*, 1990). In reproductive animals such a stimulus activates all CDCs simultaneously (Ter Maat *et al.*, 1986). This massive simultaneous discharge of activity is brought about by chemical as well as electrical transmission among the CDCs (Ter Maat *et al.*, 1988). Preliminary experiments in our laboratory have shown that electrical stimulation of a single CDC (on one side of the brain) of postreproductive animals causes a simultaneous afterdischarge in the CDCs on both sides of the brain. Moreover, depolarizing afterpotentials (see above) could still be recorded from other CDCs of postreproductive animals when a single CDC was stimulated electrically. Obviously there is still communication between the CDCs of both sides. Hence, cessation of female reproductive activity might be explained by impairment of activation of CDCs. An alternative explanation might be that CDCs are still activated but release an amount of hormone insufficient to induce egg laying. However, the properties of the afterdischarge of old non-laying snails (see above) seem to be in favour of the hypothesis that activation of CDCs is impaired in old non-laying snails.

Suppression of the electrical activity in CDCs has been reported in starved snails and in snails kept in fouled water (Ter Maat *et al.*, 1982, 1983). In starved snails the membrane potential of the CDCs is hyperpolarized and this is probably due to inhibition. As a result the cells are prevented from entering the active state (Ter Maat *et al.*, 1982). The membrane potential of CDCs of old non-reproducing snails did not differ from the other groups of snails (Janse *et al.*, 1990). Thus the lack of activity in the CDCs of old non-reproducing animals is probably not effectuated, as in starved snails, through inhibition. Possibly it is the input to the CDCs that is impaired in old non-reproducing snails.

Lymnaea can live several months after cessation of reproduction (see, for example Fig. 1). This implies that in old *Lymnaea* CDCs can be inactive for a considerable period of time. It is known that neurons degenerate when they are not actively used. Morphological studies indeed showed that in old non-laying *Lymnaea* degeneration of CDCs occurs (Joosse, 1964; Janse *et al.*, 1987b).

In addition to the changes reported above, immunocytochemical studies suggested that peptide contents of CDCs change with age. CDCs of young *Lymnaea* showed enkephalin-like immunoreactivity. In *Lymnaea* of intermediate age, the CDCs showed enkephalin-like and gastrin/cholecystokinin-like immunoreactivity. Old *Lymnaea*, however, showed only gastrin/cholecystokinin-like immunoreactivity in their CDCs (Gesser and Larsson, 1985). It is known that secretory products of the CDCs are of importance for synchronization of electrical activity in the CDC system (Ter Maat *et al.*, 1988). How age-related changes in peptide contents in CDCs relate to changes in reproductive activity of *Lymnaea* is unknown.

From the description above it is clear that with age a complex of changes in neuroendocrine organs and their targets occur. Many of the age-related changes found in the neuroendocrine system controlling reproduction seem to be of secondary origin.

Changes in peptidergic neurons with a putative role in control of cardiorespiratory functions

Although at present cardiorespiratory functions have not been studied in *Lymnaea* of different age, changes have been found in peptidergic neurons which have a putative function in cardiorespiratory control (van der Wilt *et al.*, 1987, 1988; Kerkhoven *et al.*, 1991). The neurons involved are VD1 and RPD2 which are two giant electrotonically coupled peptidergic neurons located in the visceral and right parietal ganglion, respectively (Fig. 4). VD1 and RPD2 branch extensively in the CNS and the peripheral nerves. Moreover, they send many fine fibres to the connective tissue sheath of the CNS where they form a fine network. Figure 4A shows the main branching pattern of the cells as revealed with immunocytochemical methods and with Lucifer Yellow fillings.

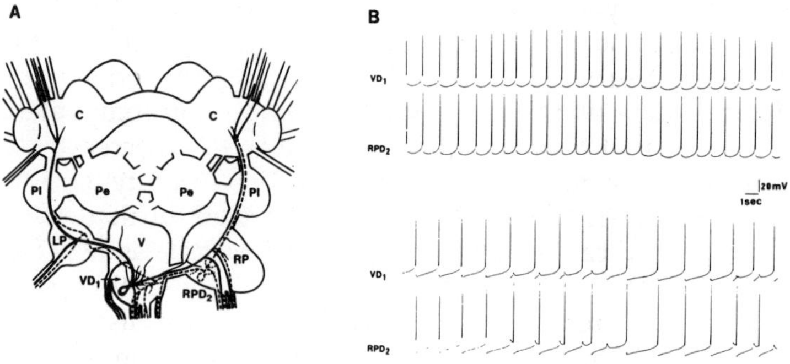

FIG. 4. A. Schematic diagram of the CNS of *Lymnaea* with branching pattern of VD1 and RPD2. B. Simultaneous intracellular recordings of VD1 and RPD2 in young (3 months) (upper two recordings) and old (12 months) (lower two recordings) *Lymnaea*. Note the disturbances in firing synchrony of the two cells in the lower pair of recordings. C: cerebral ganglion, Pe: pedal ganglion, Pl: pleural ganglion, LP and RP: left and right parietal ganglion, V: visceral ganglion (From Janse and Joosse, 1989).

Neurophysiological studies showed that both neurons receive input from oxygen-sensitive receptors in the mantle and lung area (Janse *et al.*, 1985). Taken with the extensive branching pattern of the cells, this led us to the idea that the neurons probably play an important more general role in the regulation of processes which are affected by the respiratory condition of the animal. This seems to be in line with studies on the nature of the peptide contents of the cells. With immunocytochemical methods it has been demonstrated that the cells contain an ACTH-like peptide (Boer *et al.*, 1979). Recent molecular biological studies showed that the cells are capable of synthesizing a number of peptides including peptides which show homology with those found in R15 of *Aplysia* (Boogerd *et al.*, 1991). In *Aplysia*, the contents of R15 has been shown to influence osmoregulation (Kupfermann and Weiss, 1976).

Recent observations revealed that, in addition to common synaptic input, VD1 and RPD2 each receive separate synaptic input (de Vlieger *et al.*, 1992). Integration of the different inputs of the two neurons is probably mediated by the electrical junction between the neurons. In addition it has been shown that VD1 contains a pace maker that controls the activity of the cell pair and that the junction between the cells plays an important role in the efficacy of the pace maker (Wildering, 1992; Wildering and Janse, 1992; Wildering *et al.*, 1991b). The junction is located in the left parieto-visceral connective (Benjamin and Pilkington, 1986). Normally, the neurons indeed fire their action potentials in close synchrony (Janse *et al.*, 1986b).

With age, VD1 and RPD2 increase their diameter (Janse *et al.*, 1986b). Such a neuronal growth has also been observed in other molluscs (Rattan and Peretz, 1981). Growth of the neurons is accompanied by a decrease of the input resistance (Janse *et al.*, 1986b). A decrease in input resistance generally results in a decrease in sensitivity to synaptic input. However, pharmacological experiments showed that sensitivity to histamine application in VD1 and RPD2 increases with age (Wildering *et al.*, 1992). This may mean that the expected growth-related decrease in sensitivity of the cells has been compensated for (but see Wildering, 1992 for a more detailed discussion).

In addition to the changes reported above, recent experiments (Wildering *et al.*, 1991a) indicate that active membrane properties of VD1 and RPD2 change with age. Moreover, a number of integrative properties change, resulting in a change of the firing characteristics of the neurons (Janse *et al.*, 1986b, 1987a; Wildering *et al.*, 1991; Wildering, 1992). Figure 4B shows the firing pattern of the neurons in young and old animals. One of the changes observed concerned the effectiveness of the electrical junction between the cells. The coupling efficiency of the neurons decreases considerably with age, probably due to an increase of the junctional resistance between the neurons (Janse *et al.*, 1986). Recent studies confirmed this, but also showed that in animals of 16 to 20 months of age the junction between the two cells is as effective as in young animals. Moreover, in old animals individual variance is less, probably due to an increase of mortality in animals with a high junctional resistance (Wildering *et al.*, 1991a). These data suggest that VD1 and RPD2 may be essential for survival. This is in line with the idea stated above that the cells are probably involved in regulation of processes dependent on the respiratory condition of the animal and that communication between the cells is necessary for integration of the different inputs on the two cells.

Aging in identified non-peptidergic neurons

In *Lymnaea stagnalis,* several aspects of identified giant non-peptidergic neurons have been studied by Frolkis *et al.* (1984) and Nagy *et al.* (1985). For three different types of neurons, the authors reported in older animals a decrease in excitability, a decrease in firing frequency and a decrease in velocity of repolarization of the action potential. Moreover, they found an increase in the sensitivity of the neurons to acetylcholine, norepinephrine and serotonin (Frolkis *et al.,* 1984). No changes in membrane potential were found in *Lymnaea* neurons with age (Frolkis *et al.,* 1984). In still another type of neuron the authors reported an increase of the membrane potential and an increase of the intracellular K^+-concentration (Nagy *et al.,* 1985). Obviously, not all neurons in *Lymnaea* show changes in membrane potential with age. In our laboratory we also observed that age-related changes may differ in different neurons (see below and also Janse *et al.,* 1991).

Frolkis *et al.* (1984) also studied ultrastructural aspects of *Lymnaea* neurons. They reported disintegration of cell organelles in neurons of old snails. In a more detailed study, Papka *et al.* (1981) reported an increase in lipofuscinic material in a giant identified neuron of *Aplysia.* It is known that in the molluscan CNS, lipofuscin accumulation with age depends on feeding conditions (Winstanley and Pentreath, 1985). It is, however, not known whether the presence of lipofuscin affects the functioning of neurons.

So far no studies have been done in *Lymnaea* on age-related changes in the functioning of receptors and their coupling to intracellular messenger systems. In *Mytilus,* this aspect has been studied on unidentified neurons (Stefano and Janse, 1990). Pharmacological studies showed that in this species interactions of endogenous opioids, dopamine and serotonin are involved in central regulation of ciliary beat. Increases of opioid levels were found with age, together with decreases in sensitivity of the CNS to these drugs. Probably the changes found in the CNS compensate for each other's effects on ciliary beat. Because opioids regulate dopamine release and dopamine acts on the ciliary beat, it is believed that in the intact animal the age-related changes will diminish the regulatory capacity to respond to environmental changes (Stefano and Janse, 1990). These studies demonstrate that in molluscan neurons, and probably therefore also in *Lymnaea* neurons, age-related changes and secondary compensatory changes can occur at different levels of synaptic transduction mechanisms.

Aging and nervous plasticity

One of the conspicuous features of the aging brain both in higher animals and in man is a decrease of plasticity. This is expressed as a diminished ability of learning and memory capacity and a diminished capacity to compensate functionally for brain damage (Cotman and Schiff, 1979; Drachman, 1983; McWilliams, 1988).

In molluscs, several aspects of nervous plasticity have been studied in relation to age. In *Aplysia,* it has been demonstrated that simple forms of learning decrease with age (Bailey *et al.,* 1983). In *Lymnaea,* association of food with a chemostimulus is affected by age. Old animals need to be starved to learn the association, whereas young animals can learn the association when well fed, although they also need to be starved to express the learned ability (Audesirk *et al.,* 1982). These findings are of special interest because in these animals much is known about the neuronal substrates of these functions (Bailey *et al.,* 1983; Benjamin, 1983; Mpitsos and Lukowiak, 1985; Hawkins, 1987). Thus these systems might provide an opportunity to study fundamental mechanisms underlying age-related impairment of learning and memory.

Still another aspect of plasticity of the molluscan nervous system is the capacity to restore functional connections. Peretz and coworkers showed in *Aplysia* that the width of the synaptic cleft of the neuromuscular synapses and the integrative functions of these synapses changed with age. They demonstrated that restoration of connections occurred in the old animal after a period of increased sensory input. This demonstrates that restoration of function can occur in the old molluscan nervous system (Peretz *et al.,* 1984; Peretz and Zolman, 1987; Zolman and Peretz, 1987).

In *Lymnaea,* regeneration studies showed that restoration of synaptic contacts takes place after disruption of nervous connections (Janse *et al.,* 1979; Benjamin and Allison, 1985). In this species it has been shown that restoration of reflex functions after damage of sensory input is impaired in old animals. It has been suggested that this is due to impairment of restoration of synaptic connections in the CNS of old animals (Janse *et al.,* 1986a). In the related pulmonate *Helisoma,* somatostatin influences axon outgrowth and synapse formation (Bulloch, 1987). Interestingly, in *Lymnaea,* peptidergic cells regulating growth contain a somatostatin-like peptide (Schot *et al.,* 1981). It is conceivable that in old *Lymnaea* levels of peptides involved in control of synapse formation decrease.

Common origin of aging processes in *Lymnaea*

Relationship between age-related neuronal and neuroendocrine changes

According to one of the prominent aging theories, age-related changes in the CNS may have an endocrine origin (Finch, 1976, 1988; Finch *et al.*, 1984; Landfield, 1987; Sapolsky *et al.*, 1986). If this also holds for the *Lymnaea* CNS, then a relationship could exist between reproductive endocrine changes and changes in neuronal properties. In this view one would expect that age-related changes in neuronal properties would differ in animals which reproduce at different rates. This possibility has been studied in *Lymnaea* by using the change in junctional resistance between VD1 and RPD2 as a marker of neuronal aging.

An effective way to influence the rate of reproduction in *Lymnaea* is through the feeding regimen (Bohlken and Joosse, 1982; Dogterom *et al.*, 1984). In the feeding experiments reported above (Fig. 2), at regular time intervals for each group a number of animals was sacrificed and the junctional resistance between VD1 and RPD2 was measured. The two groups fed once per week and once per two weeks, respectively, had a very low reproductive rate as compared to the group fed *ad libitum*. As already reported above, the longest survival was found in the group of animals fed once per two weeks.

The age-related change in resistance between VD1 and RPD2 appeared not to differ significantly between the animals of the different groups (Janse *et al.*, 1991b). Obviously there is no interaction between reproductive rate and the age-related change in junctional resistance. This indicates that the age-related changes in junctional resistance between VD1 and RPD2 are not related to reproductive neuroendocrine changes during aging.

The similarity in age-related junctional changes in the different animal groups also indicates that some neural age-related changes in *Lymnaea* are independent of the feeding conditions of the animals. In vertebrates, food restriction has been reported to prolong life and to suppress age-related changes at the neuron membrane level (Levin *et al.*, 1981; Weindruch and Walford, 1988; Massoro, 1988). Recent studies showed that in vertebrates also age-related changes in neural properties can be independent of feeding conditions (Massoro, 1988; Finch quoted by Weindruch and Walford, 1988). Massoro (1988) concluded in addition that there are also a number of age-related changes of non-nervous physiological processes which are not affected by feeding conditions.

Synchrony of age-related changes in neurons of different types

It is conceivable that other factors than those involved in reproductive control change with age and have wide acting direct influences on neuronal aging in *Lymnaea*. If this were true, then one would expect that with age in different types of neurons similar changes would take place. This possibility was considered by studying age-related changes in a number of neuronal properties in different types of identified single neurons but in the same animals. The following neurons were used: RPD1, RPeD1 and LPeD1 (for nomenclature see Benjamin and Winlow, 1981). Properties were studied related to soma growth, threshold of action potential generation upon electrical stimulation and maximal velocity of repolarization.

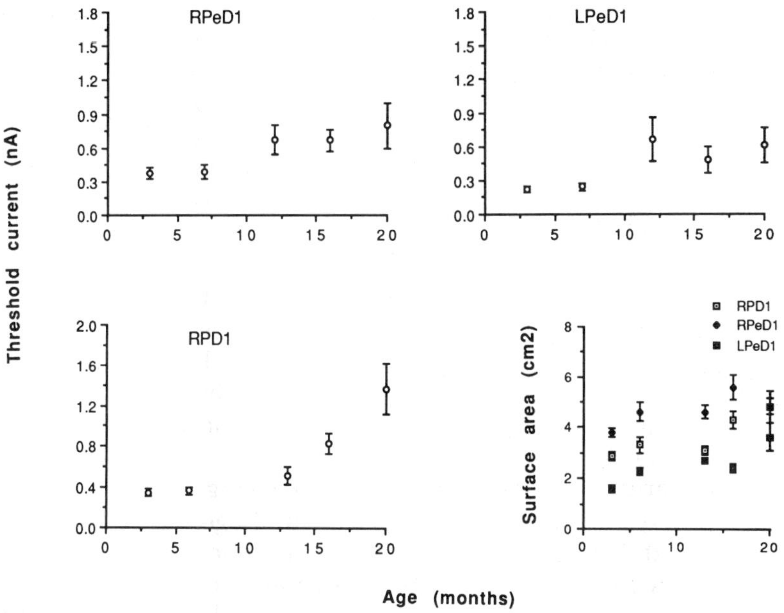

FIG. 5. Current amplitude (mean ± s.d.) needed to induce an action potential (threshold current) in different neurons as plotted against age. In all cells threshold current increased significantly with age (ANOVA, $P \leq 0.01$). Growth of the cells (calculated as indicated in Janse *et al.*, 1986b) is indicated in the lower right panel. All cells showed a significant growth with age (ANOVA, $P \leq 0.02$). $n = 7$ except in the oldest groups where $n = 4$ or 5 (From Janse *et al.*, 1991).

Figure 5 shows that threshold in the different types of neurons studied increased with age. On the other hand, however, Fig. 6 shows that the maximal velocity of repolarization (a property related to the shape of the action potential, cf. Winlow *et al.*, 1982) only changed significantly with age in RPD1. Obviously there are also particular age-related changes which differ markedly in the different neuronal types. Although the increase in cell surface with age will probably affect the electrical properties of the neurons, Figs 5 and 6 show that the changes in electrical properties cannot be fully attributed to soma growth.

The results described above suggest that some age-related changes are expressed similarly whereas others are expressed differently in different types of neurons. This implies that if there are general factors involved in neuronal aging they are differently expressed in the physiological properties of different neurons.

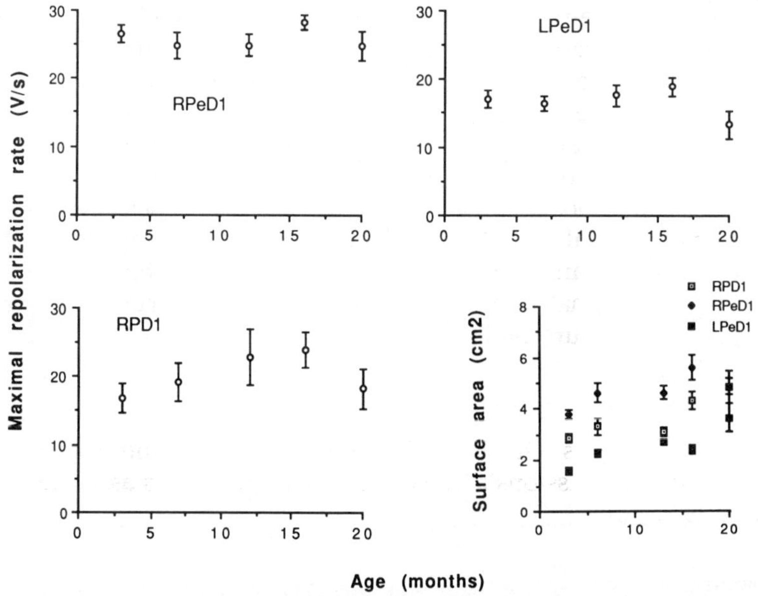

FIG. 6. Maximal repolarization rate of action potentials of different neurons (means ± s.d.) as plotted against age. Only the rate in RPD1 changed significantly with age (ANOVA, simple effects test, $P = 0.05$). See also Fig. 4.

Concluding remarks

The present study shows that in *Lymnaea* age-related changes occur at the level of the organism as well as at the neuronal level. At the organismic level age-related changes occur in important biological processes such as reproduction and growth. The changes in reproduction could be related to age-related changes at the neuronal level in nervous and neuroendocrine control mechanisms. In addition, age-related changes were found in peptidergic neurons which, putatively, control cardio-respiratory functions. The changes in the latter system seem to affect interneuronal communication. Apart from changes in peptidergic neurons, age-related changes also occur in neurons with classical transmitters.

From the present findings the picture emerges that aging is expressed widely in the CNS of *Lymnaea*. Age-related changes in different functional parts of the nervous system, however, do not necessarily show interactions. In some aspects aging is expressed similarly in different neurons, in other aspects, however, aging is, quantitatively as well as qualitatively, expressed differently. Moreover, in *Lymnaea*, feeding conditions which affect the rate of aging do not necessarily affect age-related changes at the neuronal level.

Because of the accessibility of individual neurons and the possibility to identify them from animal to animal, *Lymnaea* seems to offer a suitable model system to study age-related changes in the nervous system at the neuronal level. Moreover, these changes can be related to changes of the entire organism. On the one hand, this makes it possible to study the role of possible interactions of aging processes in different systems of the animal. On the other hand, it offers the opportunity to relate age-related changes in the nervous system to the biology of the animal. It is felt that the latter is of special importance for an understanding of (neuro)biological mechanisms of aging.

Acknowledgements

The author thanks Dr. W. C. Wildering for comments on the manuscript and discussions and M. van der Roest for his assistance in preparing the figures.

References

Adelman, R. C. and Roth, G. S. (1982). *Testing the Theories of Aging*. CRC Press, Boca Raton, Fla.

Audesirk, T. A., Alexander, J. E. Jr., Audesirk, G. J. and Moyer, C. M. (1982). Rapid, nonaversive conditioning in a freshwater gastropod. 1. Effects of age and motivation. *Behav. Neural Biol.* **36**: 379-390.

Bailey, C. H., Castellucci, V. F., Koester, J. and Chen, M. (1983). Behavioral changes in aging *Aplysia*: A model system for studying the cellular basis of age-impaired learning, memory and arousal. *Behav. Neural. Biol.* **38**: 70-81.

Benjamin, P. R. (1983). Gastropod feeding: behavioural and neural analysis of a complex multicomponent system. In: *Neural Origin of Rhythmic Movements*, eds., A. Roberts and B. Roberts, Cambridge University Press, Cambridge, pp. 159-193.

Benjamin, P. R. and Winlow, W. (1981). The distribution of three wide-acting synaptic inputs to identified neurons in the isolated brain of *Lymnaea stagnalis* (L.). *Comp. Biochem. Physiol.* **70A**: 293-307.

Benjamin, P. R. and Allison, P. (1985). Regeneration of excitatory, inhibitory and biphasic synaptic connections made by a snail giant interneuron. *Proc. R. Soc. B* **226**: 159-176.

Benjamin, P. R. and Pilkington, J. B. (1986). The electrotonic location of low-resistance intercellular junctions between a pair of giant neurons in the snail *Lymnaea*. *J. Physiol.* **370**: 111-126.

Boer, H. H., Schot, L. P. C., Roubos, E. W., ter Maat, A., Lodder, J. C., Reichelt, D. and Swaab, D. F. (1979). ACTH-like immunoreactivity in two electrotonically coupled giant neurons in the pond snail *Lymnaea stagnalis*. *Cell Tiss. Res.* **202**: 231-240.

Boer, H. H. and van Minnen, J. (1988). Immunocytochemistry of hormonal peptides in molluscs: optical and electron microscopy and the use of monoclonal antibodies. In: *Society for Experimental Biology Seminar Series, vol.* 33. *Neurohormones in Invertebrates*, eds., M. C. Thorndyke and G. J. Goldsworthy, Cambridge University Press, Cambridge, pp. 20-41.

Boer, H. H., Schot, L. P. C., Reichelt, D., Brand, H. and ter Maat, A. (1984). Ultrastructural immunocytochemical evidence for peptidergic neurotransmission in the pond snail *Lymnaea stagnalis*. *Cell Tiss. Res.* **238**: 197-201.

Bohlken, S. and Joosse, J. (1982). The effect of photoperiod on female reproductive activity and growth of the freshwater pulmonate snail *Lymnaea stagnalis* kept under laboratory conditions. *Int. J. Invert. Reprod.* **4**: 213-222.

Boogerd, J., van Kesteren, R., Veenstra, J., de Vlieger, J., Geraerts, W. P. M., van Heerikhuizen, H. and Joosse, J. (1991). Alternative splicing generates multiple variant VD1/RPD2 transcripts in the *Lymnaea* CNS. In: *Molluscan Neurobiology*, pp. 309-315, eds., K. S. Kits, H. H. Boer and J. Joosse, North Holland Publishing Co., Amsterdam.

Bulloch, A. G. M. (1987). Somatostatin enhances neurite outgrowth and electrical coupling of regenerating neurons in *Helisoma*. *Brain Res.* **412**: 6-17.

Calow, P. (1983). Life cycle patterns and evolution. In: *The Mollusca. Ecology vol. 6*, ed., W. D. Russell-Hunter, Academic Press, New York, pp. 649-678.

Capo, T. R., Perritt, S. E. and Berg, C. J. Jr. (1979). New developments in the mariculture of *Aplysia californica*. *Biol. Bull.* **157**: 360.

Comfort, A. (1957). The duration of life in Molluscs. *Proc. Mal. Soc. London* **32**: 219-241.

Comfort, A. (1979). *The Biology of Senescence.* 3rd ed., Churchill Livingstone, Edinburgh, London.

Cotman, C. W. and Schiff, S. W. (1979). Synaptic growth in aged animals. In: *Physiology and Cell Biology of Aging, vol. 8*, eds., A. Cherkin *et al.*, Raven Press, New York, pp. 109-120

Cottrell, G. A. (1977). Identified amine-containing neurones and their synaptic connections. *Neurosci.* **2**: 1-18.

Cottrell, G. A., Schot, L. P. C. and Dockray, G. J. (1983). Identification and probable role of a single neurone containing the neuropeptide *Helix*-FMRF-amide. *Nature* **304**: 638-640.

Cristofalo, V. J. (1988). An overview of the theories of biological aging. In: *Emergent Theories of Aging,* eds., J. E. Birrren and V. L. Bengston, Springer Publishing Company, New York, pp. 118-127.

De Vlieger, T. A., Wildering, W. C., van der Wolt, G. J. and Janse, C. (1992). The role of membrane properties, synaptic input and electrical junction in determination of spike output of a pair of peptidergic neurons in the mollusc *Lymnaea stagnalis. Acta Biol. Hung.* **43**(1-4): 137-146

Dogterom, G. E., van Loenhout, H., Geraerts and W. P. M. (1983). Synchronous maturation of the female reproductive system and of the ovulation hormone-producing system in *Lymnaea stagnalis. Gen. Comp. Endocr.* **52**: 242-246.

Dogterom, G. E., van Loenhout, H., Koomen, W., Roubos, E. W. and Geraerts, W. P. M. (1984). Ovulation hormone, nutritive state, and female reproductive activity in *Lymnaea stagnalis. Gen. Comp. Endocr.* **55**: 29-35.

Drachman, D. A. (1983). How normal aging relates to dementia: A critique and classification. In: *Aging of the Brain, vol. 22,* eds., D. Samuel *et al.,* Raven Press, New York, pp. 19-32.

Finch, C. E. (1976). The regulation of physiological changes during mammalian aging. *Quart. Rev. Biol.* **51**: 49-83.

Finch, C. E. (1988). Aging in the female reproductive system: A model system for analysis of complex interactions during aging. In: *Emergent Theories of Aging,* eds., J. E. Birrren and V. L. Bengston, Springer Publishing Company, New York, pp. 128-152.

Finch, C. E., Felicio, L. S., Mobbs, C. V. and Nelson, J. F. (1984). Ovarian and steroidal influence on neuroendocrine aging processes in female rodents. *Endocrine Revs.* **5**: 467-497.

Frolkis, V. V., Stupina, A. S., Martinenko, O. A., Tóth, S. and Timchenko, A. I. (1984). Aging of neurons in the mollusc *Lymnaea stagnalis*: structure, function and sensitivity to transmitters. *Mech. Ageing Dev.* **25**: 91-102.

Geraerts, W. P. M. and Joosse, J. (1975). Control of vitellogenesis and of growth of female accessory sex organs by the dorsal body hormone (DBH) in the hermaphrodite freshwater snail *Lymnaea stagnalis. Gen. Comp. Endocr.* **27**: 450-464.

Geraerts, W. P. M., Tensen, C. P. and Hogenes, Th. M. (1983). Multiple release of peptides by electrically active neurosecretory caudo dorsal cells of *Lymnaea stagnalis. Neurosci. Lett.* **41**: 151-155.

Geraerts, W. P. M., ter Maat, A. and Hogenes, Th. M. (1984). Studies on release activities of the neurosecretory caudo dorsal cells of *Lymnaea stagnalis.* In: *Biosynthesis, Metabolism and Mode of Action of Invertebrate Hormones,* eds., J. Hoffmann and M. Porchet, Springer Verlag, Berlin, pp. 44-50.

Geraerts, W. P. M., ter Maat, A. and Vreugdenhil, E. (1988). The peptidergic neuroendocrine control of egg laying behavior in *Aplysia* and *Lymnaea.* In: *Endocrinology of Selected Invertebrate Types, vol. II,* eds., H. Laufer and G. H. Downer, Liss Inc., New York, pp. 141-231.

Gesser, B. P. and Larsson, L. (1985). Changes from enkephalin-like to gastrin/cholecystokin-like immunoreactivity in snail neurons. *J. Neurosci.* **5**: 1412-1417.

Hawkins, R. D. (1987). Cellular studies of classical conditioning in *Aplysia*. In: *Neurobiology. Molluscan Models*, eds., H. H. Boer, W. P. M. Geraerts and J. Joosse, North Holland Publ. Co., Amsterdam, New York, pp. 311-319.

Hirsch, H. R. and Peretz, B. P. (1984). Survival and aging of a small laboratory population of a marine mollusc, *Aplysia californica*. *Mech. Ageing Dev.* **27**: 43-62.

Janse, C. (1974). A neurophysiological study of the peripheral tactile system of the pond snail *Lymnaea stagnalis* (L.). *Neth. J. Zool.* **24**: 93-161.

Janse, C. and Joosse, J. (1989). Ageing in molluscan nervous and neuroendocrine systems. In: *Development, Maturation and Senescence of Neuroendocrine Systems: A Comparative Approach*, eds., M. P. Schreibman and C. G. Scanes, Academic Press, New York, pp. 43-61.

Janse, C., van Beek, A., van Oorschot, I. and van der Roest, M. (1986a). Recovery of damage in a molluscan nervous system is impaired with age. *Mech. Ageing Dev.* **35**: 179-183.

Janse, C., Kits, K. S. and Lever, A. J. (1979). The re-formation of connections in the nervous system of *Lymnaea stagnalis* after nerve injury. *Mal.* **18**: 485-488.

Janse, C. , Ter Maat, A. and Pieneman, A. W. (1990). Molluscan ovulation hormone containing neurons and age-related reproductive decline. *Neurobiol. Aging* **11**: 457-463.

Janse, C., van der Roest, M. and Slob, W. (1986b). Age-related decrease in electrical coupling of two identified neurones in the mollusc *Lymnaea stagnalis*. *Brain Res.* **376**: 208-212.

Janse, C., van der Roest, M., Bedaux, J. J. M. and Slob, W. (1987a). The pond snail *Lymnaea stagnalis*, an animal model for aging studies at the neuronal level. In: *Neurobiology. Molluscan Models*, eds., H. H. Boer, W. P. M. Geraerts and J. Joosse, North Holland Publ. Co., Amsterdam, pp. 335-340.

Janse, C., Slob, W., Popelier, C. M. and Vogelaar, J. W. (1988). Survival characteristics of the mollusc *Lymnaea stagnalis* under constant culture conditions: effects of aging and disease. *Mech. Ageing Dev.* **42**: 263-274.

Janse, C., Wildering, W. C., van Minnen, J., van der Roest, M. and Roubos, E. W. (1987b). Ageing in the pond snail *Lymnaea stagnalis*. *Proc. 28th Dutch Fed. Meeting 239.*

Janse, C., Wildering, W. C. and Popelier, C. M. (1989). Age-related changes in female reproductive activity and growth in the mollusc *Lymnaea stagnalis*. *J. Gerontol.* **44**: B148-155.

Janse, C., Wildering, W. C. and van der Roest, M. (1991a). Peptidergic neurons in the aging molluscan brain. In: *Comparative Aspects of Neuropeptides*, pp. 128-139, eds., G. B. Stefano and E. Florey, Manchester University Press, Manchester.

Janse, C., Wildering, W. C. and van der Roest, M. (1991). Neuroendocrine and neural aging in the pond snail *Lymnaea stagnalis*. In: *Molluscan Neurobiology*, pp. 179-185, eds., K. S. Kits, H. H. Boer and J. Joosse, North Holland Publishing Co., Amsterdam.

Janse, C., van der Wilt, G. J., van der Plas, J. and van der Roest, M. (1985). Central and peripheral neurones involved in oxygen perception in the pulmonate snail *Lymnaea stagnalis* (Mollusca, Gastropoda). *Comp. Biochem. Physiol.* **82A**: 459-469.

Joosse, J. (1964). Dorsal bodies and dorsal neurosecretory cells of the cerebral ganglia of *Lymnaea stagnalis* L. *Arch. Néerl. Zool.* **15**: 1-103.

Joosse, J. (1979). Evolutionary aspects of the endocrine system and of the hormonal control of reproduction of molluscs. In: *Hormones and Evolution*, ed., E. J. W. Barington, Academic Press, New York, pp. 119-157.

Joosse, J. (1986). Neuropeptides: Peripheral and central messengers of the brain. In: *Comparative Endocrinology: Developments and Directions*, ed., C. Ralph, Liss Inc., New York, pp. 13-32.

Joosse, J. (1988). The hormones of molluscs. In: *Endocrinology of Selected Invertebrate Types, vol. II*, eds., H. Laufer and G. H. Downer, Liss Inc., New York, pp. 89-140.

Joosse, J. and Geraerts, W. P. M. (1983). Endocrinology. In: *The Mollusca. Part I. Physiology, vol, 4*, eds., A. S. Saleudin and K. M. Wilbur, Academic Press, New York, pp. 317-406.

Joosse, J., de Vlieger, T. A. and Roubos, E. W. (1982). Nervous systems of lower animals as models, with particular reference to peptidergic neurons in gastropods. In: *Progress in Brain Research, vol, 55. Chemical Transmission in the Brain*, eds., R. M. Buijs, P. Pévet and D. F. Swaab, Elsevier, Amsterdam, pp. 379-404.

Kandel, E. R. (1976). *Cellular Basis of Behavior*, Freeman and Company, San Francisco.

Kandel, E. R. (1979). *Behavioral Biology of Aplysia*, Freeman and Company, San Francisco.

Kempf, S. C. and Willows, A. O. D. (1977). Laboratory culture of the nudibranch *Tritonia diomedea* Bergh (Tritoniidae: Opistobranchia) and some aspects of its behavioral development. *J. Exp. Mar. Biol. Ecol.* **30**: 261-276.

Kerkhoven, R. M., Croll, R. P., van Minnen, J., Bogerd, J., Ramkema, M. D., Lodder, H. and Boer, H. H. (1991). The VD1/RPD2 neuronal system in the CNS of *Lymnaea stagnalis* and homologous systems in other molluscs with particular reference to the innervation of the auricle of the heart. In: *Molluscan Neurobiology*, pp. 255-259, eds., K. S. Kits, H. H. Boer and J. Joosse. North Holland Publishing Co., Amsterdam.

Kits, K. S. (1980). States of excitability in ovulation hormone producing neuroendocrine cells of *Lymnaea stagnalis* (Gastropoda) and their relation to the egg-laying cycle. *J. Neurobiol.* **11**: 397-410.

Kirkwood, B. L. (1985). Comparative and evolutionary aspects of longevity. In: *Handbook of the Biology of Aging*, 2nd ed., eds., C. E. Finch and E. L. Schneider, Van Nostrand Reinhold, New York, pp. 27-44.

Kooijman, S. A. L. M. (1988). The von Bertalanffy growth rate as a function of physiological parameters. A comparative analysis. In: *Mathematical Ecology*, eds., T. G. Hallam, L. J. Gross and S. A. Levin, World Scientific, Singapore, pp. 1-35.

Kriegstein, A. E., Castelllucci, V. and Kandel, E. R. (1974). Metamorphosis of *Aplysia californica* in laboratory culture. *Proc. Natl. Acad. Sci. U.S.A.* **71**: 3654-3658.

Kupfermann, I. and Weiss, K. R. (1976). Water regulation by a presumptive hormone contained in identified neurosecretory cell R15 of *Aplysia*. *J. Gen. Physiol.* **67**: 113-123.

Landfield, P. W. (1987). Modulation of brain aging correlates by long-term alterations of adrenal steroids and neurally-active peptides. In: *Progress in Brain Research, vol. 72. Neuropeptides and Brain Function*, pp. 279-300, eds., E. R. de Kloet, M. Wiegant and D. de Wied, Elsevier, Amsterdam.

Levin, P., Janda, J. K., Joseph, J. A., Ingram, D. K. and Roth, G. S. (1981). Dietary restriction retards the age-associated loss of rat striatal dopaminergic receptors. *Science* **214**: 561-562.

Lints, F. A. (1985). Non-mammalian models for research on aging. *Interdisciplinary Topics in Gerontology, vol. 21*, Barger, Basel.

Maat, A. ter, Dijks, F. A. and Bos, N. P. A. (1986). *In vivo* recordings of neuroendocrine (caudo-dorsal cells) in the pond snail. *J. Comp. Physiol.* **158**: 853-859.

Maat, A. ter, Geraerts, W. P. M., Jansen, R. F. and Bos, N. P. (1988). Chemically mediated positive feedback generates long-lasting afterdischarge in a molluscan neuroendocrine system. *Brain Res.* **438**: 853-859.

Maat, A. ter, Lodder, J. C., Veenstra J. and Goldschmeding, J. T. (1982). Suppression of egg-laying during starvation in the snail *Lymnaea stagnalis* by inhibition of the ovulation hormone producing caudo-dorsal cells. *Brain Res.* **239**: 535-542.

Maat, A. ter, Lodder, J. C. and Wilbrink, M. (1983). Induction of egg-laying in the pond snail *Lymnaea stagnalis* by environmental stimulation of the release of ovulation hormone from the caudo-dorsal cells. *Int. J. Invert. Repr.* **6**: 239-247.

McWilliams, J. R. (1988). Age-related decline in anatomical plasticity and axonal sprouting. In: *Neurology and Neurobiology, vol. 36. Neural Plasticity: A Life Span Approach*, eds., T. L. Petit and G. O. Ivy, Liss Inc., New York, pp. 329-349.

Massoro, E. J. (1988). Food restriction in rodents: An evaluation of its role in the study of aging. *J. Ger.* **43**: B59-64.

Massoro, E. J., Katz, M. S. and McMahan, C. A. (1989). Evidence for the glycation hypothesis of aging from the food-restricted rodent model. *J. Ger.* **44**: B20-22.

Mitchell, D. H. and Johnson, T. E. (1984). *Invertebrate Models in Aging Research*, Boca Raton, Florida: CRC Press, Inc.

Mpitsos, G. J. and Lukowiak, K. (1985). Learning in gastropod molluscs. In: *The Mollusca, vol. 8. Neurobiology and Behavior*, ed., A. O. D. Willows, Academic Press, New York, pp. 96-268.

Murphy, A. D., Lukowiak, K. L. and Stel, W. (1985). Peptidergic modulation of patterned motor activity in identified neurons of *Helisoma*. *Proc. Natl. Acad. Sci. U.S.A.* **82**: 7140-7144.

Nagy, I. Zs., Tóth, S. and Lustyik, Gy. (1985). Verification of the membrane hypothesis of aging on the identified giant neurons of the snail *Lymnaea stagnalis* L. (Gastropoda, Pulmonata) by a combined application of intracellular electrophysiology and X-ray microanalysis. *Arch. Gerontol. Geriatr.* **4**: 53-66.

Newell, G. E. (1964). Physiological aspects of the ecology of intertidal animals. In: *Physiology of Mollusca, vol. I*, ed., K. M. Wilbur and C. M. Yonge, Academic Press, New York, pp. 59-81.

Papka, R., Peretz, B., Tudor, J. and Becker, J. (1981). Age-dependent anatomical changes in an identified neuron in the CNS of *Aplysia californica*. *J. Neurobiol.* **12**: 455-468.

Peretz, B., Romanenko, A. and Markesbery, W. (1984). Functional history of two motor neurons and the morphometry of their neuromuscular junctions in the gill of *Aplysia*: Evidence for differential aging. *Proc. Natl. Acad. Sci. U.S.A.* **81**: 4332-4336.

Peretz, B. and Zolman, J. F. (1987). Regular activation contributes to differential aging of motor neurons in *Aplysia*. In: *Neurobiology. Molluscan Models*, eds., H. H. Boer, W. P. M. Geraerts, and J. Joosse, North Holland, Amsterdam, New York, pp. 330-334.

Rattan, K. S. and Peretz, B. (1981). Age-dependent behavioral changes and physiological changes in identified neurons in *Aplysia californica*. *J. Neurobiol.* **12**: 469-478.

Rózsa, K. S. (1984). The pharmacology of molluscan neurons. *Progr. Neurobiol.* **23**: 79-150.

Roubos, E. W. (1984). Cytobiology of the ovulation-neurohormone producing caudo-dorsal cells of the snail *Lymnaea stagnalis*. *Int. Rev. Cytol.* **89**: 295-346.

Roubos, E. W. and van der Wal-Divendal, R. M. (1980). Ultrastructural analysis of peptide-hormone release by exocytosis. *Cell Tiss. Res.* **207**: 267-275.

Russell-Hunter, W. D. (1964). Physiological aspects of ecology in nonmarine molluscs. In: *Physiology of Mollusca, vol. I*, ed., K. M. Wilburand C. M. Yonge, Academic Press, New York, pp. 83-126.

Russell-Hunter, W. D. (1983). Overview: Planetary distribution of and ecological constraints upon the mollusca. In: *The Mollusca, vol. 6, Ecology*, ed., W. D. Russell-Hunter, Academic Press, New York, pp. 1-27.

Sapolsky, R. M., Krey, L. C. and McEwen, B. S. (1986). The neuroendocrinology of stress and aging: The glucocorticoid cascade hypothesis. *Endocrine Revs.* **7**: 284-301.

Scheff, S. W., Anderson, K. and DeKosky, S. T. (1984). Morphological aspects of brain damage in aging. In: *Aging and Recovery of Function in the Central Nervous System*, ed., S. W. Scheff, Plenum Press, New York, pp. 57-85.

Scheller, R. H., Jackson, J. F., McAllister, L. B., Rothman, B. S., Mayeri, E. and Axel, R. (1983). A single gene encodes multiple neuropeptides mediating a stereotyped behavior. *Cell* **32**: 7-22.

Scheerboom, J. E. M. (1978). The influence of food quantity and food quality on assimilation, body growth and egg production in the pond snail *Lymnaea stagnalis* (L.) with particular reference to the haemolymph-glucose concentration. *Proc. Kon. Ned. Akad. Wet., Series C* **81**: 184-197.

Schot, L. P. C., Boer, H. H., Swaab, D. F. and van Noorden, S. (1981). Immunocytochemical demonstration of peptidergic neurons in the central nervous system of the pond snail *Lymnaea stagnalis* with antisera raised to biological active peptides of vertebrates. *Cell Tiss. Res.* **216**: 272-291.

Schot, L. P. C., Boer, H. H. and Wijdenes, J. (1983). Localization of neurons innervating the heart of *Lymnaea stagnalis* studied immunocytochemically with anti-FMRF amide and anti-vasotocin. In: *Molluscan Neuro-endocrinology*, eds., J. Lever and H. H. Boer, North Holland Publishing Company, Amsterdam, pp. 203-208.

Slob, W. and Janse, C. (1988). A quantitative method to evaluate the quality of interrupted animal cultures in aging studies. *Mech. Ageing Dev.* **42**: 275-290.

Steen, W. J. van der, van den Hoven, N. P. and Jager, J. C. (1969). A method for breeding and studying freshwater snails under continuous water change, with some remarks on growth and reproduction in *Lymnaea stagnalis* L. *Neth. J. Zool.* **19**: 131-139.

Stefano, G. B. and Janse, C. (1990). Molluscan models in ageing studies in the central nervous system: *Mytilus* and *Lymnaea*. In: *Neurobiology of Mytilus edulis*, ed., G. B. Stefano, Manchester University Press, New York, pp. 289-308.

Van Heukelem, W. F. (1979). Aging in lower animals. In: *The Biology of Aging*, eds., J. A. Behnke, C. E. Finch and G. B. Moment, Plenum Press, New York, pp. 115-130.

Weindruch, R. and Walford, R. L. (1988). *The Retardation of Aging and Disease by Dietary Restriction*, Charles C. Thomas, Illinois.

Whim, M. D. and Lloyd, P. E. (1990). Neuropeptide cotransmitters released from an identified cholinergic motor neuron modulate neuromuscular efficacy in aplysia. *J. Neurosci.* **10**: 3313-3322.

Wildering, W. C. (1992). Synaptic plasticity in the adult pond snail *Lymnaea stagnalis*. Thesis. Vrje University.

Wildering, W. C. and Janse, C. (1992). Serotonergic modulation of junctional conductance in an identified pair of neurons in the mollusc Lymnaea stagnalis. *Brain Res.* **595**: 343-352.

Wildering, W. C., Janse, C. and de Vlieger, T. A. (1991b). The role of the pacemaker properties and synaptic input on generation and modulation of spiking activity in a pair of electrically computed peptidergic neurons. *Brain Res.* **556**: 324-328

Wendelaar Bonga, S. E. (1970). Ultrastructure and histochemistry of neurosecretory cells and neurohaemal areas in the pond snail *Lymnaea stagnalis* (L.). *Z. Zellforschung*. **108**: 190-224.

Wildering, W. C., van der Roest, M., de Vlieger, T. A. and Janse, C. (1991). Age-related changes in junctional and non-junctional conductance in two electrically coupled peptidergic neurons of the mollusc *Lymnaea stagnalis*. *Brain Res.*

Wilt, G. J. van der, van der Roest, M. and Janse, C. (1987). Neuronal substrates of respiratory behaviour and related functions in *Lymnaea stagnalis*. In: *Neurobiology. Molluscan Models*, eds., H. H. Boer, W. P. M. Geraerts and J. Joosse, North Holland, Amsterdam, pp. 292-296.

Wilt, G. J. van der, van der Roest, M. and Janse, C. (1988). The role of two peptidergic giant neurons in modulation of respiratory behaviour in the pond snail *Lymnaea stagnalis*. In: *Symposia Biologica Hungarica, vol. 36. Neurobiology of Invertebrates. Transmitters, Modulators and Receptors*, eds., J. Salanki and K. S. Rózsa, Akadémiai Kiadó, Budapest, pp. 377-386.

Winlow, W., Holden, A. V. and Haydon, P. G. (1981). Characterization of *Lymnaea* neurones by determination of action potential trajectories. *J. Exp. Biol.* **99**: 207-221.

Winlow, W. and Haydon, P. G. (1985). A behavioural and neural analysis of the locomotory system of *Lymnaea stagnalis*. *Comp. Biochem. Physiol.* **83A**: 13-21.

Winstanley, E. K. and Pentreath, V. W. (1985). Lipofuscin accumulation and its prevention by vitamin E in nervous tissue: Quantitative analysis using snail buccal ganglia as a simple model system. *Mech. Ageing Dev.* **9**: 299-307.

Wodinsky, J. (1977). Hormonal inhibition of feeding and death of *Octopus*: control by optic gland secretion. *Science* **198**: 948-951.

Zolman, J. F. and Peretz, B (1987). Motor neuronal function in old *Aplysia* is improved by long-term stimulation of the siphon/gill reflex. *Behav. Neurosci.* **101**: 524-533.

Alterations of Opioid Regulatory Mechanisms Associated with Aging

GEORGE B. STEFANO

Multidisciplinary Center for the Study of Aging, Old Westbury Neuroscience Research Institute, State University of New York/College at Old Westbury, P.O. Box 210, Old Westbury, New York 11568, U.S.A.

Introduction

It has been suggested that with the development of a highly organized central nervous system came a prolongation of life. This greater regulation of physiological and cellular activity, including metabolic, allows for the expenditure of energy without many detrimental effects to the entire organism. Within the framework of intercellular communication, e.g., the synapse, certain alterations (receptor densities, etc.) appear to come forth so as to almost form a "guide" for future observations on alterations associated with aging (Roth, 1986). The relationship between presynaptic and postsynaptic events are directly correlated. In this regard, homeostatic mechanisms maintaining the pre- and postsynaptic relationship have been shown to be open ended in contrast to a closed loop. That is, in general, concentrations of signal molecules may change along with corresponding changes of their receptors (Roth, 1986) until further changes cannot occur.

Since the discovery of endogenous opiate-like substances, numerous and ever-increasing numbers of studies have been performed which highlight the importance of these neuropeptides not only in neurobiology but in all the life sciences. Opioid substances have been shown to have diverse functions that transcend their original proposed role in nociceptive/analgesic systems. The importance of this family of compounds is highlighted even more with their discovery in invertebrates (Stefano, 1982a, 1989; Leung and Stefano, 1987). A comparative study of opioid neurobiology associated with aging events in a simpler animal, *Mytilus edulis*, may provide valuable information about this important family of neuropeptide signal molecules.

Opioid mechanisms in *Mytilus edulis*

Receptor binding studies

Opiate receptors present in the nervous tissue of *Mytilus edulis* have properties very similar to those of opiate receptors in the mammalian nervous system. In the first detailed account of opiate binding in invertebrates (Stefano *et al.*, 1980) the binding of D-Ala^2, MePhe^4, Gly(ol)^5)-enkephalin (FK 33 824), an opiate agonist, and naloxone, an antagonist, was shown to be stereospecific, saturable, reversible, and of a high affinity. In contrast, specific binding to nonneural tissues was negligible, suggesting that the opiate sites are restricted to nervous tissues. In addition, the binding of FK 33 824 to neural elements was inhibited by sodium, a process that was reversed by manganese. The binding of naloxone was enhanced twofold in the presence of a high sodium concentration and was relatively unaffected by manganese. These differential effects of ions on agonist and antagonist binding were similar to those observed in mammalian brain homogenates. The study of Stefano *et al.* (1980) also indicated that the binding sites are probably pertinacious. The same study further substantiated the ability of various opiate agonists to enhance dopamine levels in pedal ganglia as well as the ability of naloxone to block this effect. The relative affinities of these ligands for binding to the opiate site correlated closely with the binding affinities of these ligands for enhancing dopamine levels. On the basis of these findings, the authors suggested that the sites are analogous to enkephalin-type opiate receptors (Lord *et al.*, 1976). The presence of proteolytic enzymes was also suggested since the concentrations of highly stable opioid peptides required to elicit the dopamine response were lower than those for Met- or Leu-enkephalin.

In a subsequent study (Kream *et al.*, 1980), the binding profiles obtained for various opioid ligands to membrane suspensions of pedal ganglia revealed the presence of both high- and low-affinity binding sites. Etorphine, FK 33 824, and levallorphan bound noncooperatively to a class of high-affinity sites (K_d = 1-3 nM) and cooperatively to a class of low-affinity sites (K_d = 6-11 nM). Hill analysis of the cooperative sites revealed Hill coefficients of n = 2.6-3.7, indicating markedly positive homotropic cooperativity. The total density of binding sites for all ligands was approximately 160 pmol/g of protein, whereby the high-affinity component comprised approximately 34% of the total. Kinetic analysis of the binding data obtained in *M. edulis* revealed values similar to those obtained for mammalian binding analysis; it also substantiated the cooperative nature of binding to the low-affinity site. The relative potencies of a series of opiates in displacing FK 33 824 enkephalin binding to membrane suspensions of pedal ganglia were very similar to those determined for rat brain homogenates (Kream and Zukin, 1979). The opioid peptides B-endorphin > FK 33 824 > DAMA (D-Ala^2, Met^{5}enkephalinamide) were the most potent of the ligands tested. The opiate narcotics etorphine > morphine > levorphanol exhibited intermediate potencies. Again, the relative potencies of the opioids in the displacement assay correlated closely with those determined for stimulation of dopamine levels in intact animals ($r = 0.84$).

Several possible assignments were made for the two classes of opiate binding sites in the pedal ganglia (Kream *et al.*, 1980). Presently, of the possibilities discussed, the one that seems highly likely is that the classes represent pre- and postsynaptic opiate receptors. In order to examine and substantiate this hypothesis, animals were treated with the selective neurotoxin 6-hydroxydopamine (Stefano *et al.*, 1982) as previously described (Stefano *et al.*, 1976). The results of this study (Stefano *et al.*, 1982) were as follows: The dopamine content of the pedal ganglia from lesioned animals was reduced by 33% relative to that of vehicle-treated controls. Neither serotonin nor norepinephrine levels were reduced. Fluorescence micrographs of formaldehyde-treated pedal ganglia from both lesioned and control animals revealed that the neurotoxic substance at the effective dose accumulates in the synaptically-rich neuropil, and not in the cortex (nerve cell body region) of the ganglion. Thus the partial reduction in dopamine levels may reflect a nearly total loss of dopamine in terminals with essentially no change in the nerve cell bodies. High-affinity binding of FK 33 824 (2 nM) was reduced by 81% and low-affinity binding (10 nM peptide) by 43% in pedal ganglia from lesioned animals relative to that in control tissue. In addition, DAMA, B-endorphin, and etorphine failed to change the dopamine levels in the lesioned animals. Together, these results suggest that the high-affinity opiate binding sites which mediate alteration in dopamine levels are on presynaptic dopaminergic terminals.

In other studies, opioid receptors in *Mytilus* also appear to be present on a specific population of immunocytes (Stefano *et al.*, 1989a, b, c). In this regard, actions of opioids include communication among various immunocytes present in this invertebrate (Stefano *et al.*, 1989a, b; Stefano, 1989), as also noted with human granulocytes (Stefano, 1989c;). The immunocytes in *Mytilus* contain, in addition to opioid receptors, dopamine receptor binding (Stefano *et al* 1989c).

Receptor and opioid peptide localization

The localization of opioid receptors on presynaptic nerve terminals has been documented for several areas of the mammalian nervous system, including spinal cord, vagus nerve, striatum, and amygdala (for review see Stefano, 1982; Leung and Stefano, 1987). In particular, the presence of opioid binding sites has been demonstrated directly on dopaminergic terminals in both the nigrostriatal and the mesolimbic pathways. Therefore, the opioid–dopamine interactions in *M. edulis* might be expected to be quite complex if they are analogous to the mechanisms existing in mammalian neural tissues. In 1983, Stefano and Martin demonstrated that Met-enkephalin immunoreactivity was richest in an area of the pedal ganglion heavily innervated by dopaminergic fibers, thus providing anatomical evidence for the binding and presynaptic release studies mentioned earlier in this chapter.

Modulation of presynaptic dopamine release

A major mode of action of opioid compounds may be to specifically and selectively inhibit the release of dopamine (for review see Stefano, 1982; Leung and Stefano, 1987), norepinephrine and other transmitters in regions of the mammalian central and peripheral nervous system. This action may also be directly mediated by presynaptically localized opiate receptors. In pedal ganglia of *M. edulis,* as well as in neural tissues of *Octopus bimaculatus,* morphine and DAMA suppressed the potassium-stimulated release of ^{3}H-labeled dopamine, an effect blocked by naloxone (Stefano *et al.,* 1981a). The release data strongly suggests that a population of high-affinity opioid receptors is localized on dopamine terminals (see Figures 1, 2).

Adenylate cyclase

A dopamine-stimulated adenylate cyclase was pharmacologically characterized in the pedal ganglia of *M. edulis* (Stefano *et al.,* 1981b). Dopamine, epinine, and to a lesser extent apomorphine increased cAMP levels both *in vivo* and *in vitro*. The agonist-induced elevations of cAMP content were antagonized by chlorpromazine, haloperidol, fluphenazine, and to a lesser extent 2-bromo-lysergic acid. Independently, Malanga and colleagues (1972, 1980) also characterized the dopamine receptors of the gill of *M. edulis* as D_1. In addition, an opioid interaction was demonstrated with the dopamine-stimulated cyclase (Stefano *et al.,* 1981b). Etorphine, B-endorphin, DAMA and Met-enkephalin were shown to depress the stimulation of adenylate cyclase by dopamine, an effect reversible by naloxone. Etorphine- and B-endorphin-induced inhibition of cyclase activity was shown to increase with high doses; however, the inhibition caused by Met-enkephalin and DAMA did not.

Age-Associated alterations in opioid systems

Mammals

In mammals there appears to be few studies that are concerned with the alteration of opioid metabolism as a function of the aging process. In the peripheral nervous system, Govoni *et al.* (1983) reported a decrease in the content of Met-enkephalin-like material in the coeliac and superior cervical ganglia of aged male Sprague-Dawley rats. As the authors note, given the possible role of the enkephalins as presynaptic modulators in the peripheral sympathetic system, any alteration in their metabolism or neuronal interactions may have important manifestations in the alteration of this system in older organisms. Interestingly, in the spinal cord of old male Sprague-Dawley rats, Met-enkephalin immunoreactivity decreased in the cervical and thoracic portions but not in the lumbar region (see Stefano and Leung, 1987). In addition, in the thoracic region there was an increase in the number of opioid binding sites also associated with the aging process. In the thoracic region of the spinal cord the Met-enkephalin-like material decreases and opioid receptor binding density increases, results that certainly can be discussed and interpreted as providing evidence for the existence of an opioid compensatory mechanism. In this particular region of the central nervous system this "compensatory mechanism" is opposite to that reported in invertebrates (Chapman *et al.*, 1984). However, it is important to note that the rationale for both "compensatory mechanisms" can be the same, namely, homeostasis.

There is little information available concerning levels of endogenous opioids in various brain regions in older mammals. Gambert *et al.* (1980) reported that in rat hypothalamus and corpus striatum, B-endorphin immunoreactivity did not change after maturity. It was also demonstrated that in older male Sprague-Dawley rats hypothalamus levels of B-endorphin-immunoreactive material decrease whereas levels of enkephalin-like material do not change. Kumar and colleagues (1980) reported that in comparing, the Met-enkephalin levels in the hypothalamus of an old Long Evans female were not different from levels in hypothalamus of younger rats. In another study (Steger *et al.,* 1980) the Met-enkephalin content of the hypothalamus was found to be higher in old male Sprague-Dawley rats. Barden *et al.* (1981) found a decrease in the B-endorphin-immunoreactive material in particular regions of the hypothalamus of old male rats. In a more detailed study, Dupont *et al.* (1981), analyzing individual hypothalamic regions, found a decrease in Met-enkephalin-like material in the n. suprachiasmaticus, n. arcuatus, and n. premamillaris ventralis and found no changes in the other hypothalamic nuclei studied. In the same study, Leu-enkephalin-like material was found to be lower in the n. preopticus medialis, n. suprachiasmaticus, n. paraventricularis, n. ventromedialis and n. premamillaris ventralis. Tang and colleagues (1984) reported levels of Met-enkephalin as well as Met-enkephalin-Arg^6-Phe^7 in the pituitary and other brain regions of young and old male and female Sprague-Dawley rats. That study revealed higher opioid levels in the pituitary of older animals, whereas in the hypothalamus, levels were reduced markedly. Reduced Met-enkephalin levels were reported in the substantia nigra of patients dying with Parkinson's disease (Taquet *et al.*, 1982). In old male C57BL/6J mice immunoreactive B-endorphin content decreased in the neurointermediate pituitary and hypothalamus, whereas immunoreactive enkephalin decreased in the striatum and dorsolateral cortex (Rogers *et al.*, 1985). Thus, these studies serve to demonstrate that different brain regions may vary regarding opioid levels as organisms age. The results may also be a consequence of the variations in the individual scientific protocols, sex and strain of the animals, ages compared, etc. For example, in the study of Tang and colleagues (1984) 18 months was considered to be old, whereas in other studies (e.g., Dupont *et al.*, 1981) 24-26 months was considered to be old. Yet another variation in these studies is the length of the animal's light–dark cycle. The male rats were either kept on a 12- hour cycle (Tang *et al.*, 1984) or a 14-hour light–10 hour dark–cycle (Dupont *et al.*, 1981). Another potential source for variation in opioid content is the endogenous diurnal rhythm (Tang *et al.*, 1984). In the hypothalamus and striatum of adult male Sprague-Dawley rats Met-enkephalin and Met-enkephalin-Arg^6-Phe^7 were found to be higher during the dark cycle than in the light. These sources of potential variation in opioid levels also indicate that the endogenous opioid mechanisms present in the organisms are quite complex and dynamic.

Unlike the hypothalamus, the pituitary appears to exhibit a higher degree of age-related alterations. The level of Met-enkephalin-immunoreactive material increases in the pituitary of older female (Kumar *et al.*, 1980) and male rats. The level of B-endorphin-like material also was higher in the old male rats. In addition, the level of the high molecular weight opioid precursor molecules were higher in older rats. B-endorphin immunoreactivity was not examined in the old female rats (Kumar *et al.*, 1980).

Only a few studies have investigated opioid receptor mechanisms during the aging process. McDougal *et al.* (1980) demonstrated a decrease in the specific binding density of ^{3}H-naloxone in the hypothalamus of old male Fischer rats. Messing *et al* (1980, 1981), employing ^{3}H-dihydromorphine, found a decrease in the binding site densities in the striatum, anterior cortex and frontal cortices of male rats and in the midbrain and thalamus of old female Fischer 344 rats. It is of interest to note that the binding affinities were the same for all ages and sexes, with the exception of the frontal poles which were 2 × higher in the older rats. Simultaneously, Hess *et al.* (1981), employing ^{3}H-etorphine, also observed a decrease in the binding site densities in the striatum, hippocampus and frontal cortices of old male Wistar rats. Other brain regions were examined, but alterations in the binding densities as well as the affinity constant were not found. Previously it was noted that in the spinal cord of old male Sprague-Dawley rats stereoselective DAMA binding studies revealed an increase in the receptor binding densities concomitant with lower Met-enkephalin-like material. Thus, given the limited amount of information, with increasing age there appears to be a general decline in opioid receptor densities in specific brain areas. At present, data is not available regarding the influence of the aging process on opiate receptor subtypes. In addition, for the most part, the affinity of the receptor for its ligand appears not to be affected by the aging process.

In recent years attempts were made to examine alterations in pain sensitivity during the aging process (see Leung and Stefano, 1987). However, at present, the results of these studies appear to be conflicting. In mice and rats, a decrease in the sensitivity of the organisms to electrical shock has been noted, whereas others report an increase. Interestingly, in older humans narcotic placebo administration has a higher frequency of success than in younger individuals. In another study, following surgery narcotics were found to have greater analgesic actions in older humans (see Leung and Stefano, 1987).

As previously noted, in the dorsal horn region of mammals Met-enkephalin is postulated to be an important element in pain transmission. Spinal analgesia has been proposed to be related to inhibition by Met-enkephalin of substance P release from primary afferent neurons in the region of the substantia gelatinosa (Mudge *et al.*, 1979; Lamotte *et al.*, 1976; Hokfelt *et al.*, 1977). These findings have been incorporated into a functional rationale for the increased efficacy of analgesic-like compounds in geriatric patients. Namely, an increased number of receptors at the level of the dorsal horn may be available for drug–receptor interactions. In reviewing previous sections of this report, we find that in different brain regions we find differences in the expression of the endogenous opioid system with age not only with respect to receptor densities (Messing *et al.*, 1980, 1981; Hess *et al.*, 1981) but, also to levels (Dupont *et al.*, 1981; Barden *et al.*, 1981; Tang *et al.*, 1984).

At present, it is not certain to what extent age-associated alterations are associated with alterations in analgesia and perception of pain. As is widely known, pain is an extremely complex sensation. In addition, not all pain pathways/mechanisms involve opioids as the principal nociceptive agents. In opioid-mediated analgesia, the various levels at which aging alterations may occur are numerous (i.e. synthesis and degradation modifications, affinity and density of receptors, interaction with other cellular components/mechanisms, etc.). Clearly, given this level of complexity, we may find different alterations in different brain regions or disorders associated with aging. Age-associated modifications in this system may manifest themselves as additive/exponential behavioral changes. Given a particular functional priority of various brain regions, we may witness alterations which are different, yet the opioid system may be the same. Also, these alterations in the opioid system probably occurred over relatively long time periods, which leads us to the conclusion that steady state mechanisms may apply only to short time intervals within a life cycle. In the overall life, cycle homeostasis occurs, yet the underlying mechanisms retain the capacity for acute responses in order to protect an organism from sudden changes.

Invertebrates

Changes in opioid receptors and in endogenous opioids

The levels of the endogenous opioids were estimated in mussels at different ages (Chapman *et al.*, 1984; Makman and Stefano, 1984). In *Mytilus* there was a dramatic increase in the Met-enkephalin and Met-enkephalin-Arg^6-Phe^7 content from the 1-, 2- to 4-year-old animals. The change in *Mytilus* pedal ganglia amounts to a 5-fold and 10-fold increase in the levels of Met-enkephalin and Met-enkephalin-Arg^6-Phe^7, respectively. Leu-enkephalin was not detected at the time of this study due to seasonal variations, which appears to be a important factor in the expression of the endogenous opioids in this organism.

In the cerebral ganglia of the insect *Leucophaea maderae*, opioid binding sites have been demonstrated (Stefano and Scharrer, 1981). HPLC analyses of the cerebral ganglia extracts by Chapman *et al.* (1984) revealed a substance which migrates as Met-enkephalin. In this study Leu-enkephalin and Met-enkephalin-Arg^6-Phe^7 were not detected. It was quite apparent that in *Leucophaea*, as in *Mytilus*, the "Met-enkephalin" content increased dramatically during the aging process.

There was a 6-fold increase in the content of this peptide in adult organisms that were 14 months old compared to those that were 2 months old.

The binding characteristics of opioid receptors was first studied in the visceral ganglia of *Mytilus edulis* in reference to alterations with age. Specific and saturable high-affinity binding was observed for all age groups (1, 2, and 4 years old; Stefano, 1981, 1982) using ^{3}H-naloxone and ^{3}H-etorphine. Scatchard analysis revealed similar affinity constants for all age groups. In the older animals the binding site density was approximately 30% lower as compared to the younger animals. In a subsequent study, Chapman *et al.* (1984) extended the study to include the pedal ganglia of *Mytilus edulis*. The pedal ganglia of *Mytilus* contains both a high and lower affinity opioid binding site (Kream *et al.*, 1980). It was demonstrated that in the pedal ganglia for all age groups the affinity constants remain the same for both binding sites. The study also demonstrated that only the high-affinity binding site density was altered in the older organisms, being about 30% less. The binding density of the lower affinity site was not altered. The high-affinity opioid binding site density found in the insect *Leucophaea* cerebral ganglia was reduced in older organisms (Chapman *et al.*, 1984), whereas the affinity constant remained the same.

Opioid agonist binding in invertebrate neural tissues, as in vertebrate tissues, is inhibited by sodium, whereas antagonist binding is enhanced (Stefano *et al.*, 1980). In older *Mytilus* there appears to be an age-correlated decrease in the magnitude of the sodium effect on opioid binding (Chapman *et al.*, 1984). This effect has not been examined in the mammalian nervous system.

The loss of opioid binding sites is apparently correlated with a loss of dopamine responsiveness to opioid administration in older *Mytilus* (Stefano, 1981; Chapman *et al.*, 1984). These results support the hypothesis that the high-affinity opioid binding site found in the pedal ganglia of *Mytilus* is present on dopaminergic neurons (Stefano *et al.*, 1982; Stefano and Martin, 1983). Thus, there appear to be alterations in the interaction of dopamine and the endogenous opioid system with age.

The specific decrease in the high-affinity binding site density together with the corresponding increase in endogenous opioid levels in the pedal ganglia of *Mytilus* with age suggests the presence of a compensatory mechanism. This mechanism probably demonstrates the existence of a complex intercellular feedback process. There are numerous possible explanations for this compensatory mechanism; however, at the present time it is too early to speculate.

Functional alterations

Age-related changes in neuronal function are likely to be reflected in changes of specific neurotransmitter or neuromodulator systems. A large number of vertebrate neurotransmitter and neuromodulator substances are present in the same or closely analogous form in invertebrates. Recently, Aiello *et al.* (1986; Aiello and Hager, 1986) demonstrated that various opiates can modulate the central dopaminergic inhibitory mechanism associated with regulating peripheral lateral ciliary activity (Figures 1, 2). Previously, in *Mytilus*, it was demonstrated that serotonin applied to either the cerebral ganglion (for review see Aiello *et al.*, 1986), visceral ganglion or gill would cause cilioexcitation. Dopamine applied to the same tissues would cause cilioinhibition (Aiello *et al.*, 1986), thus establishing an antagonistic system in the regulation of lateral ciliary activity. In subsequent studies, these signal molecules were found to be endogenous to these tissues. These observations led to the conclusion that the visceral ganglion supplies dopaminergic, cilioinhibitory nerves to the lateral epithelium of the gill (Figure 1). A parallel series of observations indicates that the visceral ganglion also supplies the gill with a serotonergic, cilioexcitatory innervation. The studies of Aiello and colleagues (1986) also incorporate a physiological role for endogenous opioids in the regulation of dopaminergic activity. Briefly, dopamine applied to the Cerebral ganglion inhibited lateral ciliary activity. This effect can be blocked by applying opioids to the visceral ganglion, which is situated in the cerebral–gill neural pathway. This blockade of dopamine cilioinhibition by opiates can be reversed by the opiate antagonist naloxone. In preparations with low endogenous rates of ciliary beating, the beating rate was stimulated by opiates, an effect reversed by naloxone. Preparations with high endogenous rates were inhibited by naloxone addition to the visceral ganglion. From these studies and others noted in that report, it was postulated that the cilioinhibitory, dopaminergic mechanism includes nerves running from the cerebral ganglion to the gill with synaptic transmission in the visceral ganglion that can be modulated by endogenous opioids. The mechanism involved is believed to be the presynaptic inhibition of dopamine release by endogenous opioid peptides (Figure 2). Opioids applied to the visceral ganglion would inhibit dopamine release, effectively blocking the cilioinhibitory mechanism. Therefore, the cilioexcitation caused by opiates would be due to unmasking or allowing the 5-HT system to operate freely.

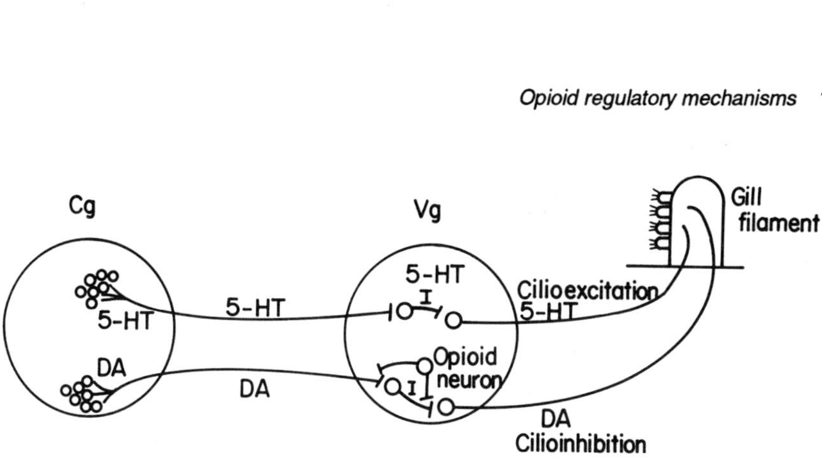

FIG. 1. Dual innervation of lateral ciliated cells in the gill of *Mytilus edulis*. Serotonergic (5-HT) and dopaminergic (DA) neurons that innervate the lateral ciliated epithelium of the gill may originate from the cerebral ganglia (Cg). The vast majority of these fibers appear to innervate other neurons [possible interneurons (I)] in the visceral ganglia (Vg). Evidence also indicates that there may be a lower percent of fibers that pass directly through the Vg to innervate, in part, the gill (not shown). The Vg also appears to have neurons that send fibers directly to the lateral ciliated cell. Furthermore, it is believed that endogenous opioid peptides may modulate the release of dopamine by way of an opioid interneuron. The end functional result of these pathways is that 5-HT stimulation causes cilioexcitation and dopamine causes cilioinhibition. However, opioid peptides by blocking the release of dopamine also would allow for cilioexcitation. Indeed the ciliated cells may be kept in an inhibited state pending opioid activity which would disinhibit these cells indirectly at the Vg. See text for specific experiments and discussion.

In regard to aging, only the visceral ganglion cilioexcitatory response to serotonin was altered, in that older animals were unable to achieve the higher ciliary beating rates obtained in younger animals (Stefano *et al.*, 1987) (Figure 2). The dopaminergic ciliary inhibitory response was also examined in preparations with a high endogenous rate of beating. Younger organisms were found to have higher endogenous rates of beating. Also, in older animals only one in twenty-five preparations exhibited beats above 900, whereas this rate was exceeded by over 70% in young animals. Older animals were more sensitive to dopaminergic inhibition since ciliary beating stopped at a lower dose of dopamine applied to the ganglia. However, dopamine was found to exert the same effect when applied to the gill, indicating a ganglionic alteration associated with aging rather than a peripheral one. Thus far, the data indicate that in older organisms a stronger inhibitory influence, in regard to regulating the rate of ciliary beating, is present. To further test this hypothesis the following experiments were performed. Since etorphine had previously been shown to inhibit dopamine release in the visceral ganglia (Stefano *et al.*, 198la), and thereby to allow for cilioexcitation (Aiello *et al.*, 1986), we tested its ability to enhance cilioexcitation in older animals. Animals are grouped according to age and also according to initial ciliary activities. It has been consistently found in previous studies that the endogenous rate in freshly opened mussels varies considerably and unpredictably from one animal to the next and it has been proposed that one explanation for this would be the existing level of endogenous enkephalinergic modulation of the DA system (Aiello *et al.*, 1986). The results of the present study are consistent with this explanation.

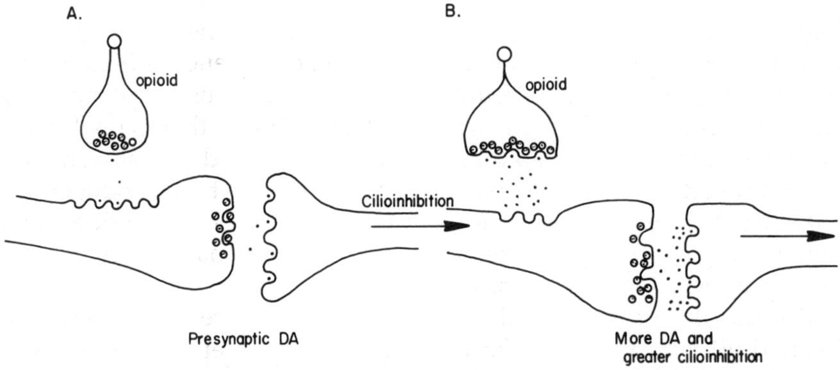

FIG. 2. Alteration of the opioid modulation of presynaptic dopamine release associated with aging. A. In younger *Mytilus* endogenous opioid peptides appear to regulate the presynaptic release of dopamine. That is, opioid peptides inhibit the release of dopamine. Physiologically, this can be observed indirectly by noting the ciliary beating rates (see Figure 1 and text). B. In older organisms there appears to be higher intraganglionic opioid peptide levels associated with a decrease in the opioid binding density without a change of the receptor affinity constant. Physiologically, one would expect the beating of the cilia on the lateral cells to be lower, given the greater presence of dopamine, the cilioinhibitory signal molecule, since the opioid "system" appears to be diminishing in its functional capacity. This is just what has been found, older organisms have lower endogenous ciliary beating rates. See text for specific experiments and discussion.

Young animals selected for low initial beating rates showed higher average rates of beating than old animals and are less likely to be totally quiescent and attain faster rates when stimulated with serotonin. Etorphine activates quiescent cilia and accelerates beating cilia in both groups, with the younger animals achieving a higher beating rate. The strong activation of the older animals by etorphine indicates that the inhibition of dopamine release was occurring. Since etorphine does not have a serotonin-like effect when added directly to the gill, its activity on the visceral ganglion is presumably due to its enkephalin-like action (Aiello *et al.*, 1986). The conclusion is that low beating rates in these animals is due to dopaminergic activity, with relatively little enkephalinergic activity, especially in older animals (Figure 2). Old animals are capable of rapid beating but at a lower rate than young animals. Interestingly, when the beating is extremely high, etorphine has no effect. Presumably, at these maximal rates serotonin is operating alone, as would be expected if there were no dopaminergic activity in these animals or if dopaminergic neurons had been blocked in the visceral ganglia by endogenous enkephalin (Figures 1, 2). Experiments differentiating the effects of naloxone on high and maximal beating rates indicate that when beat frequency is high it may indeed be due to the suppression of endogenous dopamine by endogenous enkephalinergic activity. It was shown that (1) naloxone does not have a direct inhibitory action of its own and (2) naloxone has a cilioinhibitory effect upon blocking the effect of endogenous enkephalin, only if there is a significant level of endogenous dopaminergic activity. Therefore, older animals may be controlled more predominantly by dopamine.

Because the effector in this system is the lateral cell of the gill, the isolated gill was examined for differences in endogenous activity and sensitivity to serotonin and dopamine (Stefano *et al.*, 1987). In the absence of the central nervous system, these differences indicate that the endogenous rate of autonomous beating also varies from animal to animal. There is no age-related difference in either endogenous rates or the effects of serotonin and dopamine on the non-innervated gill. However, when the visceral ganglia is attached, the older animals have lower rates and the magnitude of the response at a high level of serotonin is less. The responses to dopamine were comparable in old and young animals. Since input from the cerebral ganglia is not present, it suggests that there is more dopaminergic or less serotonergic activity originating in the visceral ganglion. This could be because of a lower influence of the endogenous enkephalinergic activity in older animals.

Consistent with this possibility, the ability of etorphine to suppress the K^+-stimulated release of dopamine was found to be reduced in older animals (Stefano *et al.*, 1987). In younger organisms the total radioactivity released and attributed to the etorphine inhibition of dopamine release is approximately 7% of the total ganglionic content as opposed to 3.7% in the older animals' visceral ganglia. Thus, there appears to be a significant reduction in the response of the dopamine release mechanism to opioids in older animals (Figure 2B). The stimulation of dopamine release by KCl is identical for all age groups, suggesting the specificity of the reduced sensitivity.

In order to further test the hypothesis that dopaminergic cilioinhibition is enhanced in older organisms and that this inhibitory enhancement is located in the visceral ganglion, the ganglion was treated with the neurotoxin 6-hydroxydopamine. Previously, this agent was shown to selectively destroy DA terminals at this dose in *Mytilus* (Stefano *et al.*, 1976, 1982). In both young and older organisms the endogenous beating rate was higher when compared to vehicle treated controls and there was no difference in the endogenous beating rate between the two groups of animals. Thus, the results indicated that in older organisms dopaminergic cilioinhibition becomes more prominent, probably due to enhanced dopamine release which can be accounted for by a decreased presynaptic responsiveness to endogenous opioids (Figure 2B).

The "key" alteration in this neuropeptide–biogenic amine interaction may reside in the regulation of synthesis of the peptide gene products, e.g., a derepression of regulating synthesis. Clearly, this is a complicated problem and many interpretations of the data are possible. Given the striking similarities of the opioid–dopamine interaction in both mammals and molluscs (Stefano, 1982a; Leung and Stefano, 1987; Stefano *et al.*, 1992), it is of interest to speculate that the aging alterations noted in this report may also have counterparts in mammals. Clearly, the interaction between these two signal systems has been maintained through the course of evolution relatively intact (Stefano, 1986, 1991).

Conclusions

Age-associated alterations in opioid activities can have profound affects on an organism's ability to survive. The significance of this family of compounds can be noted by their presence in practically all physiological systems as well as being present in diverse animals. Interestingly, the homeostasis within opioid expression and transduction to biological action at a receptor appears to change in an animal's life span. At present, it can only be surmised that the alteration associated with this homeostasis is detrimental to an overall functional or dynamic capacity to survive and cope with both external and internal "forces" that further stress opioid mechanisms.

Acknowledgements

The author wishes to thank the many collaborators and students who worked on the numerous projects outlined in this review, for without their help this area of scientific endeavor could not have progressed to the point it has. During the preparation of the manuscript the author was partially supported by Grant MH/DA 47392, ADAMHA-MARC Grant 17138, The Long Island Community Foundation, Inc., Hoffmann LaRoche Pharmaceuticals, and The Upjohn Company.

References

Aiello, E., Hager, E., Akiwumi, C. and Stefano, G. B. (1986). An opioid mechanism modulates central and not peripheral dopaminergic control of ciliary activity in the marine mussel *Mytilus edulis*. *Cell. Mol. Neurobiol.* **6**: 17-30.

Aiello, E. and Hager, E. (1986). An opioid mechanism modulates dopaminergic control of ciliary activity in the marine mussel *Mytilus edulis*. In: *Comparative Opioid and Related Neuropeptides*, Vol. II. ed., G. B. Stefano. Boca Raton, Florida, CRC Press.

Barden, N., Dupont, A., Labrie, F., Meraud, Y., Rouleau, D., Vaudry, H. and Boissier, J. R. (1981). Age dependent changes in the B-endorphin content of discrete brain nuclei. *Brain Res.* **208**: 209-212.

Chapman, A., Gonzales, G., Burrowes, W. R., Assanah, P., Iannone, B., Leung, M. K. and Stefano, G. B. (1984). Alterations in high-affinity binding characteristics and levels of opioids in invertebrate ganglia during aging: evidence for an opioid compensatory mechanism. *Cell. Mol. Neurobiol.* **4**: 143-155.

Dupont, A., Savard, P., Merand, Y., Labrie, F. and Boissier, J. R. (1981). Age-related changes in central nervous system enkephalins and substance P. *Life Sci.* **29**: 2317-2322.

Gambert, S. R., Garthwaite, T. L., Pontzer, C. H. and Hagen, T. C. (1980) Age-related changes in central nervous system beta-endorphin and ACTH. *Neuroendocrinology* **31**: 252-255.

Govoni, S., Missale, C., Castelletti, L., Spano, P. F. and Trabucchi, M. (1983). Decreased content of met-enkephalin-like peptides in superior cervical and coeliac ganglia of aged rats. *Neurobiol. Aging* **4**: 147-150.

Hess, G. D., Joseph, J. A. and Roth, G. S. (1981). Effect of age on sensitivity to pain and brain opiate receptors. *Neurobiol. Aging* **2**: 49-55.

Hokfelt, T., Ljungdahl, A., Terenius, L., Elde, R. and Wilsson, G. (1977). Immunohistochemical analysis of peptide pathways possibly related to pain and analgesia: Enkephalin and substance P. *Proc. Natl. Acad. Sci. USA.* **74**: 3081-3085.

Kream, R. M. and Zukin, R. S. (1979). Binding characteristics of a potent enkephalin analog. *Biochem. Biophys. Res. Commun.* **90**: 99-109.

Kream, R. M., Zukin, R. S. and Stefano, G. B. (1980). Demonstration of two classes of opiate binding sites in the nervous tissue of the marine mollusc *Mytilus edulis*. *J. Biol. Chem.* **225**: 9218-9224.

Kumar, M. S. A., Chen, C. L. and Huang, H. H., (1980). Pituitary and hypothalamic concentration of met-enkephalin in young and old rats. *Neurobiol. Aging* **1**: 153-155.

Lamotte, C., Pert, C. B. and Snyder, S. H. (1976). Opiate receptor binding in primate spinal cord: Distribution and changes after dorsal section. *Brain Res.* **112**: 567-568.

Leung, M. K. and Stefano, G. B. (1987) Comparative neurobiology of opioids with special attention to senescent alterations. *Prog. in Neurobiol.* **28**: 131-159.

Lord, J. A. H., Waterfield, A. A., Hughes, J. and Kosterlitz, H. W. (1976). Multiple opiate receptors. In: *Opiates and Endogenous Opioid Peptides,* ed., H. W. Kosterlitz, North-Holland, Amsterdam, Elsevier, pp. 275-280.

Makman, H. H. and Stefano, G. B., (1984). Marine mussels and cephalopods as models for study of neuronal aging. In: *Invertebrate Models in Aging Research,* eds., D. H. Mitchell and T. E. Johnson, Boca Raton, Fl, CRC Press. pp. 165-189.

Malanga, C. J., Wenger, G. R. and Aiello, E. (1972). Endogenous dopamine in bivalve gills. *Comp. Biochem. Physiol.* **43A**: 825-830.

Malanga, C. J., Poll, K. A. and O'Donnell, J. P. (1980). Agonist and antagonist effects of dopaminergic stimulation of cAMP in the ciliated cell epithelium of the marine mussel *Mytilus edulis. Fed. Proc.* **29**(3): Abstr. 3179.

McDougal, J. N., Pedigo, N. W., Marques, P. R., Vamamura, H. I. and Burks, T. F. (1980). Opiate binding characteristics in senescent rats. *Abstracts of the Society of Neuroscience* **6**: 78.

Messing, R. B., Vasquez, B. J., Spiehler, V. R., Martinez, J. L., Jensen, R. A., Righter, H. and McGaugh, J. L. (1980). ^{3}H-dihydromorphine binding in brain regions of young and old aged rats. *Life Sci.* **26**: 921-927.

Messing, R. B., Vasquez, B. J., Samaniego, B., Jensen, R. A., Martinez, J. L. and McGaugh, J. L. (1981). Alterations in dihydromorphine binding in cerebral hemispheres of aged male rats. *J. Neurochem.* **36**: 784-790.

Mudge, A. W., Leeman, S. E. and Fischbach, G. D. (1979). Enkephalin inhibits release of substance P from sensory neurons in culture and decreases action potential duration. *Proc. Natl. Acad. Sci. USA.* **76**: 526.

Rogers, J., Shoemaker, W. J., Morgan, D. G. and Finch, C. E. (1985) Senescent change in tissue weight and immunoreactive B-endorphin, enkephalin and vasopressin in eight regions of C57BL/6J mouse brain and pituitary. *Neurobiol. of Aging* **6**: 1-9.

Roth, G. S. (1986). Altered biochemical responsiveness and hormone receptor changes during aging. In: *The Biology of Aging.* eds., J. A. Behnke, C. E. Finch and G. A. Moment. Plenum Press, New York, pp. 291-300.

Stefano, G. B., Catapane, E. J. and Aiello, E. (1976). Dopaminergic agents influence serotonin in molluscan nervous system. *Science* **194**: 539-541.

Stefano, G. B., Kream, R. M. and Zukin, R. S. (1980). Demonstration of stereospecific opiate binding in the nervous tissue of the marine mollusc *Mytilus edulis. Brain Res.* **181**: 445-450.

Stefano, G. B. (1981). Decrease in the number of high affinity opiate binding sites during the aging process in *Mytilus edulis* (Bivalvia). *Cell. Mol. Neurobiol.* **4**: 343-350.

Stefano, G. B. and Scharrer, B. (1981). High affinity binding of an enkephalin analog in the cerebral ganglion of the insect *Leucophaea maderae* (Blattaria). *Brain Res.* **225**: 107-114.

Stefano, G. B., Hall, B., Makman, M. H. and Dvorkin, B. (1981a). Opioids inhibit potassium-stimulated dopamine release in the marine mussel *Mytilus edulis* and the cephalopod *Octopus bimaculatus. Science* **213**: 928-930.

Stefano, G. B., Catapane, E. J. and Kream, R. M. (1981b). Characterization of the dopamine-stimulated adenylate cyclase in the pedal ganglia of *Mytilus edulis*: interactions with etorphine, B-endorphin, DALAa and methionine enkephalin. *Cell. Mol. Neurobiol.* **1**: 57-68.

Stefano, G. B. (1982a). Comparative aspects of opioid–dopamine interaction. *Cell. Mol. Neurobiol.* **2**: 167-178.

Stefano, G. B. (1982b). Aging: variations in opiate binding characteristics and dopamine responsiveness in subtidal and intertidal *Mytilus edulis* visceral ganglia. *Comp. Biochem. Physiol.* **72C**: 349-352.

Stefano, G. B., Zukin, R. S. and Kream, R. M. (1982). Evidence for the presynaptic localization of a high affinity opiate binding site on dopamine neurons in the pedal ganglia of *Mytilus edulis* (Bivalvia). *J. Pharmacol. Exp. Ther.* **222**: 759-764.

Stefano, G. B. and Martin, R. (1983). Enkephalin-like immunoreactivity in the pedal ganglion of *Mytilus edulis* (Bivalvia) and its proximity to dopamine containing structures. *Cell. Tissue Res.* **230**: 147-153.

Stefano, G. B. (1986). Conformational matching: A possible evolutionary force in the evolvement of signal system. In: *Comparative Opioid and Related Neuropeptide Mechanisms, vol. 2,* ed., G. B. Stefano, Boca Raton, Florida, USA, CRC Press.

Stefano, G. B., Braham, E., Finn, P., Aiello, E. and Leung, M. K. (1987) Aging alterations in the modulation of central dopaminergic cilioinhibition by etorphine in the marine mussel, *Mytilus edulis*: Decrease in the inhibition of presynaptic dopamine release. *Cell. Mol. Neurobiol.* **7**: 209-219.

Stefano, G. B. and Leung, M. K. (1986). Opioid aging and seasonal variation in invertebrate ganglia: Evidence for an opioid compensatory mechanism. In: *Comparative Opioid and Related Neuropeptide Mechanisms, vol. 2,* ed., G. B. Stefano, Boca Raton, Florida, USA, CRC Press.

Stefano, G. B. (1989). Role of opioid neuropeptides in immunoregulation. *Prog. in Neurobiol.* **33**: 149-159.

Stefano, G. B., Zhao, X., Bailey, D., Metlay, M. and Leung, M. K. (1989a) High affinity dopamine binding to mouse thymocytes and *Mytilus edulis* (Bivalvia) hemocytes. *J. Neuroimmunology* **21**(1): 67-74.

Stefano, G. B., Leung, M. K., Zhao, X. and Scharrer, B. (1989b). Evidence for the involvement of opioid neuropeptides in the adherence and migration of immunocompetent invertebrate hemocytes. *Proc. Natl. Acad. Sci. USA* **86**: 626-630.

Stefano, G. B., Cadet, P. and Scharrer, B. (1989c). A novel neuropeptide receptor demonstrated in invertebrate immunocytes by opioid induced cellular responses. *Proc. Natl. Acad. Sci. USA* **86**: 6307-6311.

Stefano, G. B. (1991). Conformational matching a stabilizing signal system factor during evolution: additional evidence in comparative neuroimmunology. *Adv. Neuroimmunol.* **1**: 71-82.

Stefano, G. B., Melchiorri, P., Negri, L., Hughes, T. K. and Scharrer, B. (1992). (D-Ala^2)-deltorphin I binding and pharmacological evidence for a special subtype of delta opioid receptor on human and invertebrate immune cells. *Proc. Natl. Acad. Sci. USA* **89**: 9316-9320.

Steger, R. W., Sonntag, W. E., Van Vugt, D. A., Forman, L. J. and Meites, J. (1980). Reduced ability of naloxone to stimulate LH and testosterone release in aging male rats: possible relation to increase in hypothalamic met-enkephalin. *Life Sci.* **27**: 747-753.

Tang, F., Tang, J., Chou, J. and Costa, E. (1984). Age-related and diurnal changes in met-enkephalin-Arg-Phe and met-enkephalin contents of pituitary and rat brain structures. *Life Sci.* **35**: 1005-1014.

Taquet, H., Javoy-Agid, F., Cesselin, F., Hamon, M., Legrand, J. C. and Agid, Y. (1982). Microtopography of methionine, enkephalin, dopamine and noradrenaline in the ventral mesencephalon of human control and Parkinsonian brains. *Brain Res.* **235**(2): 303-314

SUBJECT INDEX